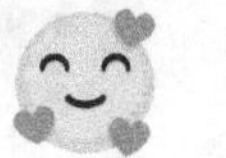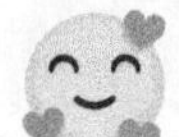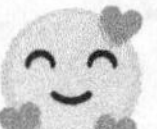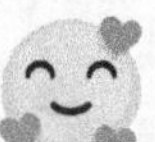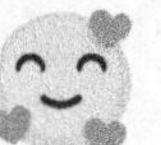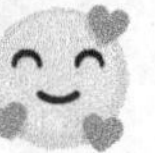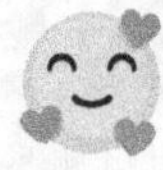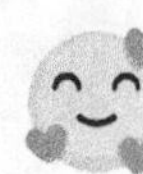

2. Overnight Chia Pudding with Almond Milk

Let's do that and fill in the time here

 Prep Time :   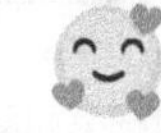 Cook Time :   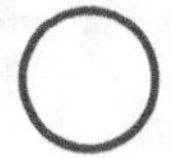 Servings :

Write 5 friends with whom you want to share this dish

....

....

....

....

....

INGREDIENTS

- 1/4 cup chia seeds
- 1 cup unsweetened almond milk
- 1 tbsp honey or maple syrup (optional)
- 1/2 tsp vanilla extract
- Pinch of cinnamon
- Fresh berries, nuts, or other toppings (optional)

Is this dish easy or difficult for you to make?

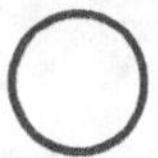 ◯   ◯

1. In a medium-sized bowl or mason jar, combine the chia seeds, almond milk, honey/maple syrup (if using), vanilla extract, and cinnamon. Stir well to combine.

2. Cover the bowl or seal the mason jar and refrigerate overnight or for at least 4 hours, until the chia seeds have absorbed the liquid and the pudding has thickened.

3. Before serving, give the pudding a good stir to break up any clumps. Top with fresh berries, nuts, or other desired toppings.

This chia pudding is a great option for a menopausal diet for several reasons:

1. Chia seeds are a good source of fiber, protein, and omega-3 fatty acids, which can help support overall health and potentially alleviate some menopausal symptoms.

2. Almond milk is a dairy-free, low-calorie, and nutrient-rich alternative to cow's milk, which can be beneficial during menopause.

3. The optional honey or maple syrup provides a touch of sweetness without using refined sugar, which can be helpful for managing blood sugar levels.

4. The fresh berries and nuts add additional fiber, vitamins, and healthy fats to the dish.

How would you rate this dish?

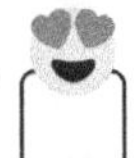 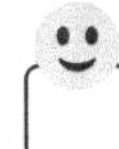  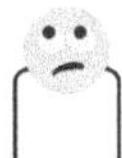 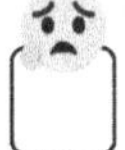

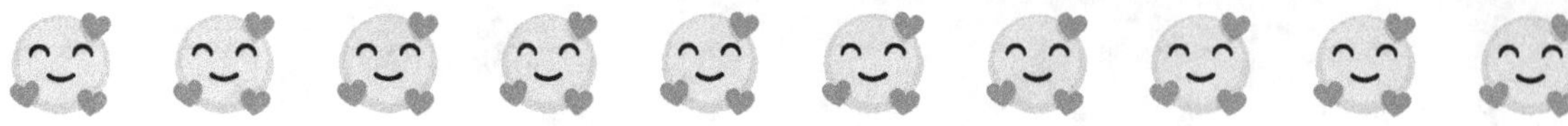

3. Oatmeal with Fresh Fruits and Nuts

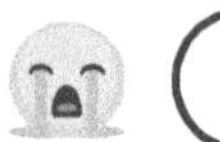 Prep Time :

Cook Time :

Servings :

Write 5 friends with whom you want to share this dish ....

Is this dish easy or difficult for you to make?

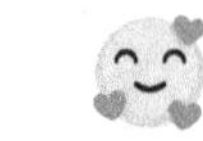 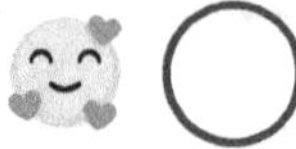

INGREDIENTS

- 1 cup old-fashioned rolled oats
- 1 1/2 cups unsweetened almond milk (or milk of your choice)
- 1 tbsp honey or maple syrup (optional)
- 1/2 tsp ground cinnamon
- 1/4 cup mixed fresh berries (such as blueberries, raspberries, and/or sliced strawberries)
- 2 tbsp chopped walnuts or almonds

1. In a medium saucepan, combine the rolled oats and almond milk. Bring the mixture to a simmer over medium heat, stirring occasionally.

2. Reduce the heat to low and continue to cook the oatmeal, stirring frequently, until it reaches your desired thickness, about 5-7 minutes.

3. Remove the oatmeal from the heat and stir in the honey or maple syrup (if using) and the ground cinnamon.

4. Transfer the oatmeal to a bowl and top with the fresh berries and chopped nuts.

This oatmeal dish is a great option for a menopausal diet for several reasons:

1. Oats are a complex carbohydrate that can help provide sustained energy and support heart health during menopause.

2. The fresh berries are rich in antioxidants, fiber, and vitamins, which can help support overall health and potentially alleviate some menopausal symptoms.

3. The nuts, such as walnuts or almonds, provide healthy fats, protein, and fiber, which can help promote feelings of fullness and support bone health.

4. The optional honey or maple syrup provides a touch of sweetness without using refined sugar, which can be helpful for managing blood sugar levels.

How would you rate this dish?

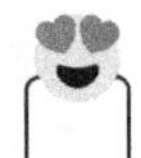 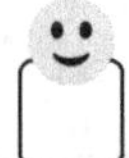 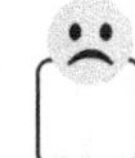 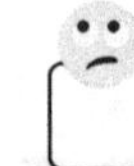 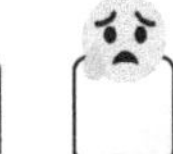

Welcome to ***"The Good Food Menopause Diet Cookbook: A Comprehensive Guide to Flavorful Meals That Alleviate Menopause Symptoms and Promote Well-being."*** This book is designed to be your trusted companion on a journey through one of the most significant transitions in a woman's life—menopause. It's a time of change, both physically and emotionally, but it's also a time when you can take charge of your health and well-being like never before.

Menopause is a natural part of aging, but its symptoms—hot flashes, night sweats, mood swings, and weight gain, to name a few—can be challenging. The good news is that what you eat can have a profound impact on how you feel. By choosing the right foods, you can alleviate many of the uncomfortable symptoms and improve your overall health.

This cookbook is more than just a collection of recipes; it's a guide to understanding the powerful role that nutrition plays during menopause. We'll explore how certain foods can help balance hormones, boost energy levels, and support your body through this transformative time. You'll find information on key nutrients, practical tips for meal planning, and delicious recipes that are easy to prepare and packed with flavor.

Each recipe in this book has been carefully crafted to provide maximum nutritional benefits while tantalizing your taste buds. Whether you're looking for hearty breakfasts, satisfying lunches, nourishing dinners, or guilt-free desserts, you'll find plenty of options to suit your needs and preferences.

In the chapters ahead, we'll delve into:

- ***Understanding Menopause:*** Learn about the hormonal changes that occur during menopause and how they affect your body.

- ***The Power of Nutrition:*** Discover the essential nutrients that can help manage menopause symptoms and support overall health.

- ***Smart Eating Strategies:*** Get practical advice on meal planning, portion control, and mindful eating to make the most of your menopause diet.

- ***Delicious Recipes:*** Enjoy a wide variety of recipes that are not only nutritious but also bursting with flavor, from breakfasts and smoothies to main courses and snacks.

Our goal is to empower you with the knowledge and tools to make informed choices about your diet, so you can feel your best during menopause and beyond. Embrace this new chapter with confidence, knowing that you have the resources to nourish your body and enhance your well-being.

Thank you for joining us on this journey. Let's get cooking and start feeling great!

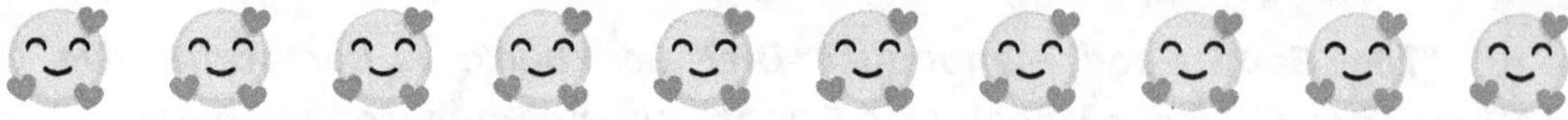

1. Greek Yogurt with Berries and Flaxseeds

 *Let's do that and fill in the time here* Prep Time : 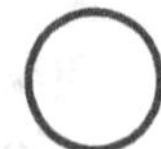 Cook Time : 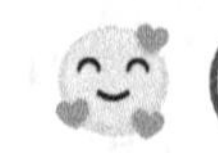 Servings :

Write 5 friends with whom you want to share this dish

....

....

....

....

....

Is this dish easy or difficult for you to make?

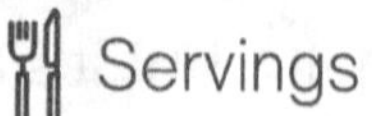 

INGREDIENTS

- 1 cup plain Greek yogurt
- 1/2 cup mixed berries (such as blueberries, raspberries, and/or strawberries)
- 1 tbsp ground flaxseeds

1. Spoon the Greek yogurt into a bowl.

2. Top the yogurt with the mixed berries.

3. Sprinkle the ground flaxseeds over the top.
4. Enjoy!

This recipe is a great option for a menopausal diet for a few reasons:

1. Greek yogurt is an excellent source of protein, which can help maintain muscle mass and bone health during menopause.

2. Berries are rich in antioxidants, fiber, and vitamins, which can help support overall health and potentially alleviate some menopausal symptoms.

3. Flaxseeds are a good source of fiber, omega-3 fatty acids, and phytoestrogens, which may help with some menopausal symptoms.

This simple, nutrient-dense snack or breakfast can be a great addition to a balanced menopausal diet. Let me know if you have any other questions!

How would you rate this dish?

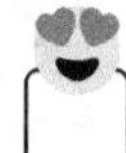 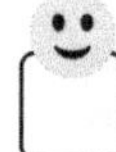 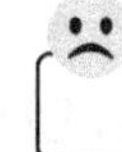 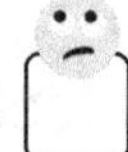 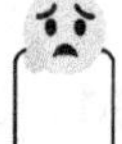

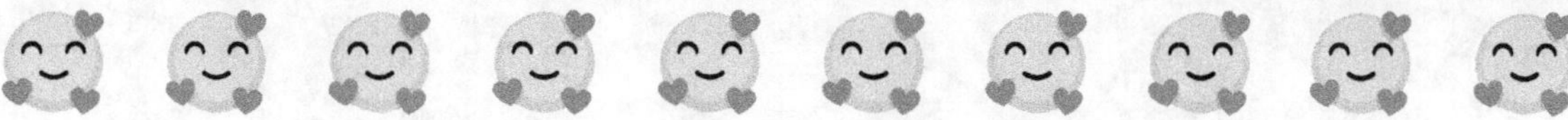

4. Avocado Toast with Whole Grain Bread

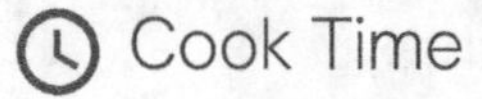 Prep Time :   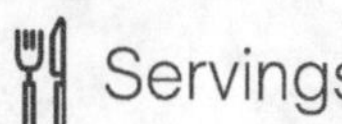 Cook Time :   Servings :

Is this dish easy or difficult for you to make?

 ◯   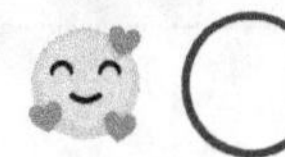 ◯

Write 5 friends with whom you want to share this dish

....

....

....

....

....

INGREDIENTS

- 2 slices of whole grain or sprouted bread
- 1 ripe avocado, mashed
- 1 tbsp lemon juice
- 1/4 tsp garlic powder (optional)
- Salt and pepper to taste
- Toppings (optional): sliced tomatoes, radishes, microgreens, or a drizzle of olive oil

1. Toast the whole grain or sprouted bread slices until lightly golden.

2. In a small bowl, mash the avocado with the lemon juice, garlic powder (if using), and a pinch of salt and pepper.

3. Spread the mashed avocado evenly over the toasted bread slices.

4. Top the avocado toast with any desired toppings, such as sliced tomatoes, radishes, or microgreens. Drizzle a small amount of olive oil over the top, if desired.

This avocado toast is a great option for a menopausal diet for several reasons:

1. Whole grain or sprouted bread provides complex carbohydrates, fiber, and nutrients that can help support overall health during menopause.

2. Avocado is a rich source of healthy monounsaturated fats, which can help promote feelings of fullness and support heart health.

3. The lemon juice and optional garlic powder add flavor and potential anti-inflammatory benefits.

4. The toppings, such as tomatoes, radishes, and microgreens, provide additional vitamins, minerals, and antioxidants that can support overall health during menopause.

This easy and versatile breakfast or snack can be a great addition to a balanced menopausal diet.

How would you rate this dish?

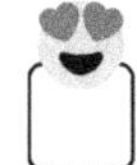  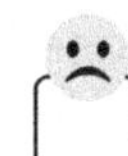 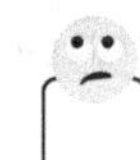 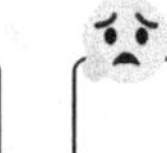

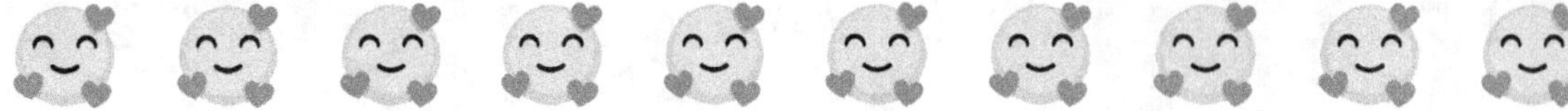

5. Smoothie with Spinach, Banana, and Protein Powder

 Prep Time :   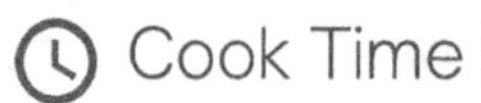 Cook Time :   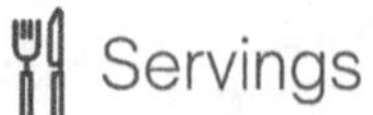 Servings :

Write 5 friends with whom you want to share this dish

....

....

....

....

....

Is this dish easy or difficult for you to make?

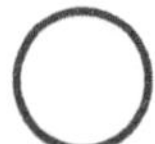 ◯   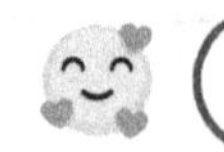 ◯

INGREDIENTS

- 1 cup unsweetened almond milk (or milk of your choice)
- 1 cup fresh spinach leaves
- 1 ripe banana, frozen
- 1 scoop of unflavored or vanilla protein powder (such as whey, pea, or plant-based protein)
- 1 tbsp ground flaxseeds (optional)
- 1 tsp honey or maple syrup (optional)

1. In a high-speed blender, combine the almond milk, spinach, frozen banana, protein powder, and ground flaxseeds (if using).

2. Blend the ingredients on high speed until the mixture is smooth and creamy, about 1-2 minutes.

3. Taste the smoothie and add a teaspoon of honey or maple syrup if you'd like it to be slightly sweeter.

4. Pour the smoothie into a glass and enjoy immediately.

This spinach, banana, and protein powder smoothie is a great option for a menopausal diet for several reasons:

1. Spinach is a nutrient-dense leafy green that provides a variety of vitamins, minerals, and antioxidants that can support overall health during menopause.

2. Bananas are a good source of potassium, which can help regulate blood pressure and potentially alleviate some menopausal symptoms.

3. Protein powder helps to provide a boost of high-quality protein, which can help maintain muscle mass and support bone health during menopause.

4. The optional ground flaxseeds are a good source of fiber, omega-3 fatty acids, and phytoestrogens, which may help with some menopausal symptoms.

This smoothie can be a quick and easy way to incorporate a variety of nutrient-dense ingredients into your menopausal diet.

How would you rate this dish?

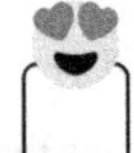 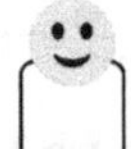 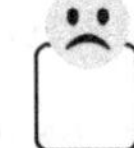 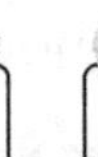 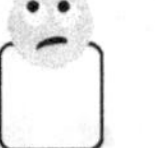 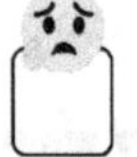

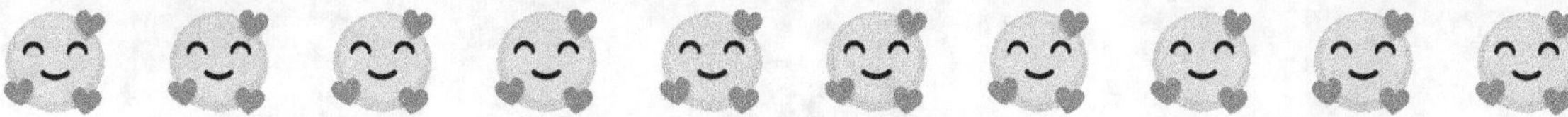

6. Scrambled Eggs with Spinach and Tomatoes

 Prep Time :   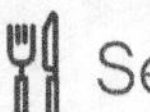 Cook Time :   Servings :

Is this dish easy or difficult for you to make?

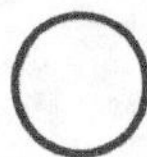 ◯   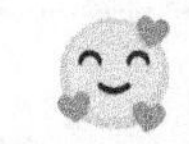 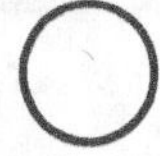 ◯

Write 5 friends with whom you want to share this dish

....

....

....

....

....

INGREDIENTS

- 3 large eggs
- 1 tbsp unsweetened almond milk (or milk of your choice)
- 1 cup fresh spinach leaves, chopped
- 1/2 cup cherry or grape tomatoes, halved
- 1 tsp olive oil
- Salt and pepper to taste

4. The dish is low in carbohydrates and high in protein and healthy fats, which can help regulate blood sugar levels and promote feelings of fullness.

This quick and easy scrambled egg dish can be a great addition to a balanced menopausal diet.

1. In a small bowl, whisk together the eggs and almond milk until well combined.

2. Heat the olive oil in a non-stick skillet over medium heat.

3. Add the chopped spinach to the skillet and cook for 1-2 minutes, until slightly wilted.

4. Pour the egg mixture into the skillet and use a spatula to gently scramble the eggs, incorporating the spinach as you go.

5. Once the eggs are almost fully cooked, add the halved tomatoes to the skillet and continue to cook for another 1-2 minutes, until the eggs are fully set and the tomatoes are slightly softened.

6. Season the scrambled eggs with salt and pepper to taste. Serve the scrambled eggs with spinach and tomatoes immediately.

This scrambled egg dish is a great option for a menopausal diet for several reasons:

1. Eggs are an excellent source of high-quality protein, which can help maintain muscle mass and support bone health during menopause.

2. Spinach is a nutrient-dense leafy green that provides a variety of vitamins, minerals, and antioxidants that can support overall health during menopause.

3. Tomatoes are a good source of lycopene, an antioxidant that may help reduce the risk of certain health conditions associated with menopause.

How would you rate this dish?

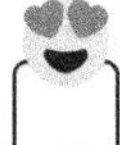 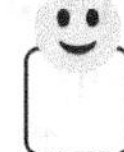 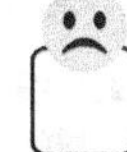 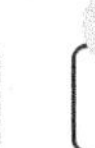 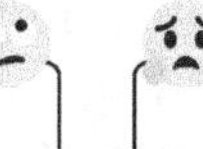

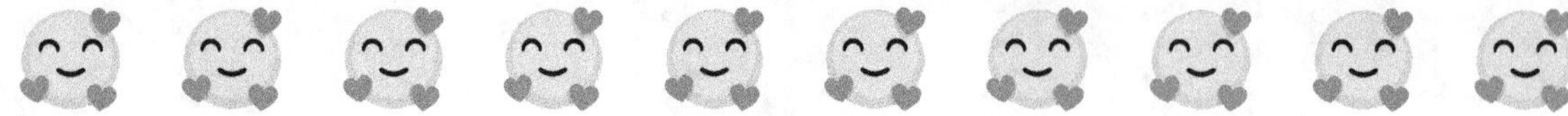

7. Quinoa Breakfast Bowl with Almonds and Blueberries

 Prep Time : 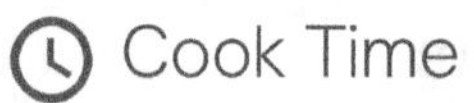 Cook Time : 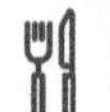 Servings :

Is this dish easy or difficult for you to make?

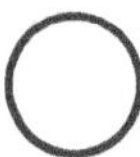 ◯   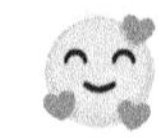 ◯

Write 5 friends with whom you want to share this dish

....

....

....

....

....

INGREDIENTS

- 1/2 cup cooked quinoa, cooled
- 1/2 cup unsweetened almond milk
- 1/4 cup fresh or frozen blueberries
- 2 tbsp sliced almonds
- 1 tsp honey or maple syrup (optional)
- Pinch of cinnamon

1. In a medium bowl, combine the cooked quinoa and almond milk. Stir to combine.

2. Top the quinoa mixture with the fresh or frozen blueberries, sliced almonds, and a drizzle of honey or maple syrup (if using).

3. Sprinkle a pinch of cinnamon over the top. Enjoy the quinoa breakfast bowl warm or chilled.

This quinoa breakfast bowl is a great option for a menopausal diet for several reasons:

1. Quinoa is a nutrient-dense whole grain that provides complex carbohydrates, protein, and fiber, which can help support sustained energy and feelings of fullness during menopause.

2. Blueberries are rich in antioxidants, vitamins, and fiber, which can help support overall health and potentially alleviate some menopausal symptoms.

3. Almonds are a good source of healthy fats, protein, and fiber, which can help promote feelings of fullness and support bone health during menopause.

4. The optional honey or maple syrup provides a touch of sweetness without using refined sugar, which can be helpful for managing blood sugar levels.

5. Cinnamon is a spice that may have anti-inflammatory properties and can potentially help regulate blood sugar levels.

This versatile and nutrient-dense breakfast can be a great addition to a balanced menopausal diet.

How would you rate this dish?

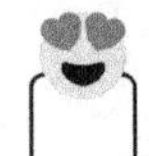 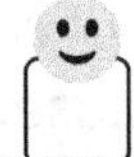 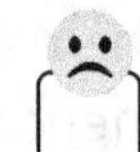 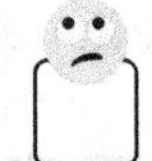 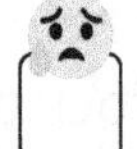

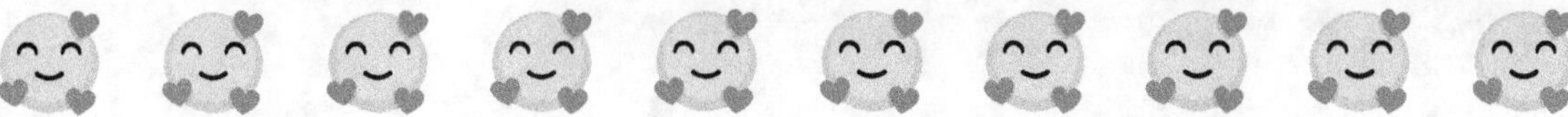

8. Cottage Cheese with Pineapple and Chia Seeds

 Prep Time :    Cook Time :   Servings :

Is this dish easy or difficult for you to make?

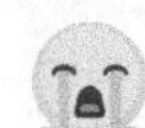  ◯   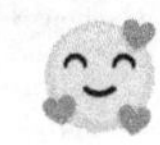 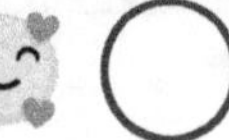 ◯

Write 5 friends with whom you want to share this dish

....
....
....
....
....

INGREDIENTS

- 1 cup low-fat or non-fat cottage cheese
- 1/2 cup fresh or canned pineapple chunks
- 1 tbsp chia seeds
- 1 tsp honey (optional)

1. In a small bowl, combine the cottage cheese, pineapple chunks, and chia seeds.

2. If desired, drizzle the honey over the top and stir gently to combine.

3. Enjoy the cottage cheese mixture immediately or refrigerate until ready to serve.

This cottage cheese dish is a great option for a menopausal diet for several reasons:

1. Cottage cheese is an excellent source of protein, which can help maintain muscle mass and support bone health during menopause.

2. Pineapple is a good source of vitamin C, which can help support immune function and potentially alleviate some menopausal symptoms.

3. Chia seeds are a rich source of fiber, omega-3 fatty acids, and antioxidants, which can help promote overall health and potentially alleviate some menopausal symptoms.

4. The optional honey provides a touch of sweetness without using refined sugar, which can be helpful for managing blood sugar levels.

This simple and versatile dish can be enjoyed as a snack or a light meal, and it can be a great addition to a balanced menopausal diet.

How would you rate this dish?

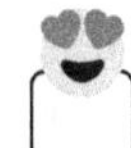 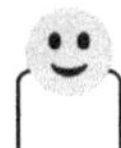 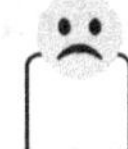 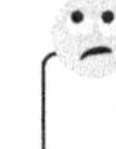 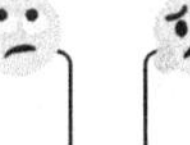 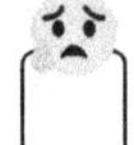

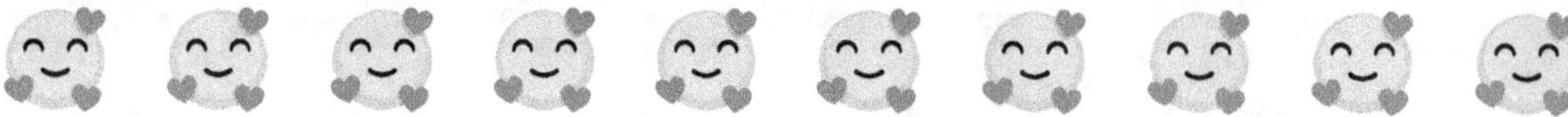

9. Banana Pancakes with Oats and Eggs

 Prep Time :  Cook Time : Servings :

Is this dish easy or difficult for you to make?

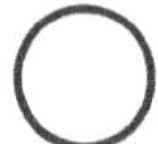 ⭕  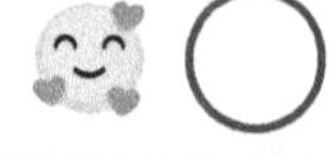 ⭕

Write 5 friends with whom you want to share this dish

INGREDIENTS

- 1 ripe banana, mashed
- 2 large eggs
- 1/2 cup old-fashioned rolled oats
- 1 tsp baking powder
- 1/4 tsp ground cinnamon
- Pinch of salt
- Coconut oil or butter for cooking

1. In a medium bowl, mash the ripe banana until smooth.

2. Add the eggs and whisk together until well combined.

3. Stir in the rolled oats, baking powder, cinnamon, and a pinch of salt. Mix until the ingredients are just combined (do not overmix).

4. Heat a non-stick skillet or griddle over medium heat and lightly grease with coconut oil or butter.

5. Scoop the batter onto the hot surface, using about 1/4 cup of batter per pancake.

6. Cook the pancakes for 2-3 minutes per side, or until golden brown.

7. Serve the banana pancakes warm, with your choice of toppings such as fresh berries, a drizzle of honey, or a sprinkle of chopped nuts.

These banana pancakes are a great option for a menopausal diet for several reasons:

1. Bananas are a good source of potassium, which can help regulate blood pressure and potentially alleviate some menopausal symptoms.

2. Oats are a complex carbohydrate that can provide sustained energy and support heart health during menopause.

3. Eggs are an excellent source of high-quality protein, which can help maintain muscle mass and support bone health.

How would you rate this dish?

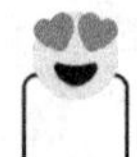 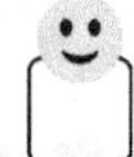 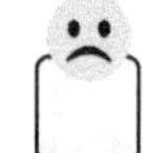 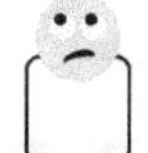 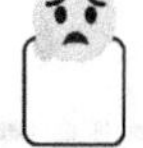

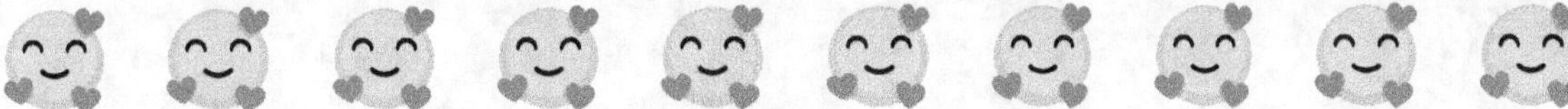

10. Whole Grain Muffins with Walnuts and Carrots

 Prep Time : 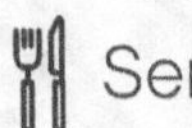 Cook Time : Servings :

Is this dish easy or difficult for you to make?

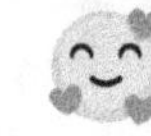 ◯   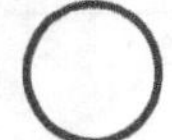 ◯

Write 5 friends with whom you want to share this dish

....

....

....

....

....

INGREDIENTS

- 1 cup whole wheat flour
- 1/2 cup old-fashioned oats
- 1 tsp baking powder
- 1/2 tsp baking soda
- 1/4 tsp ground cinnamon
- 1/4 tsp salt
- 2 large eggs
- 1/2 cup unsweetened applesauce
- 1/4 cup honey or maple syrup
- 1 tsp vanilla extract
- 1 cup grated carrots
- 1/2 cup chopped walnuts

1. Preheat your oven to 375°F (190°C). Grease a 12-cup muffin tin or line it with paper liners.

2. In a medium bowl, whisk together the whole wheat flour, oats, baking powder, baking soda, cinnamon, and salt.

3. In a separate bowl, beat the eggs. Then stir in the applesauce, honey or maple syrup, and vanilla extract.

4. Pour the wet ingredients into the dry ingredients and mix just until combined. Fold in the grated carrots and chopped walnuts.

5. Divide the batter evenly among the prepared muffin cups, filling them about 3/4 full.

6. Bake for 18-20 minutes, or until a toothpick inserted into the center comes out clean.

7. Allow the muffins to cool in the tin for 5 minutes before transferring them to a wire rack to cool completely.

These whole grain muffins are a great option for a menopausal diet for several reasons:

1. Whole wheat flour and oats provide complex carbohydrates, fiber, and nutrients that can help support sustained energy and overall health during menopause.

2. Carrots are a good source of beta-carotene, which can have antioxidant properties and potentially alleviate some menopausal symptoms.

How would you rate this dish?

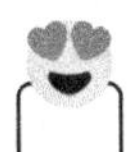 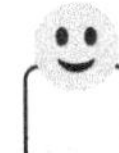 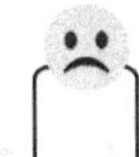 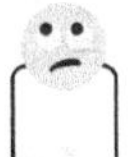 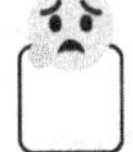

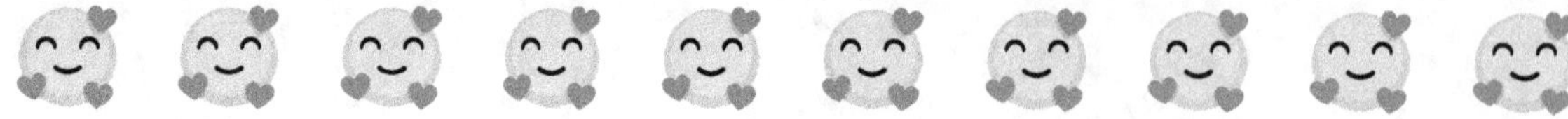

11. Grilled Chicken Salad with Mixed Greens and Avocado

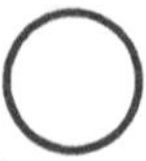 Prep Time :   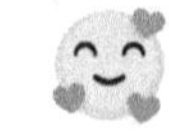 Cook Time :   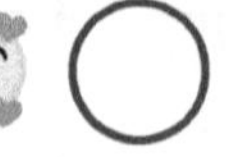 Servings :

Write 5 friends with whom you want to share this dish

....
....
....
....
....

Is this dish easy or difficult for you to make?

 ◯   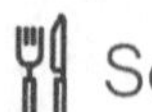 ◯

INGREDIENTS

- 4 oz grilled chicken breast, sliced
- 4 cups mixed greens (such as spinach, arugula, and kale)
- 1/2 avocado, sliced
- 1/4 cup cherry tomatoes, halved
- 2 tbsp sliced almonds
- 1 tbsp olive oil
- 1 tbsp balsamic vinegar
- 1 tsp Dijon mustard
- Salt and pepper to taste

1. In a large salad bowl, combine the mixed greens, sliced grilled chicken, avocado slices, cherry tomatoes, and sliced almonds.

2. In a small bowl, whisk together the olive oil, balsamic vinegar, and Dijon mustard to make the dressing.

3. Drizzle the dressing over the salad and toss gently to coat.

4. Season the salad with salt and pepper to taste. Serve the grilled chicken salad immediately.

This grilled chicken salad is a great option for a menopausal diet for several reasons:

1. Grilled chicken is an excellent source of lean protein, which can help maintain muscle mass and support bone health during menopause.

2. Mixed greens, such as spinach, arugula, and kale, are nutrient-dense and provide a variety of vitamins, minerals, and antioxidants that can support overall health during menopause.

3. Avocado is a rich source of healthy monounsaturated fats, which can help promote feelings of fullness and support heart health.

4. The cherry tomatoes and almonds add additional fiber, vitamins, and healthy fats to the salad.

5. The balsamic vinegar and Dijon mustard in the dressing provide a flavorful way to add healthy fats and reduce the need for added sugars.

How would you rate this dish?

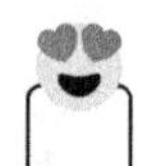 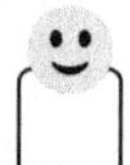  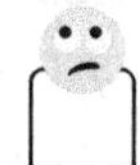 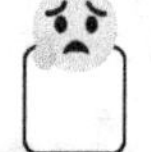

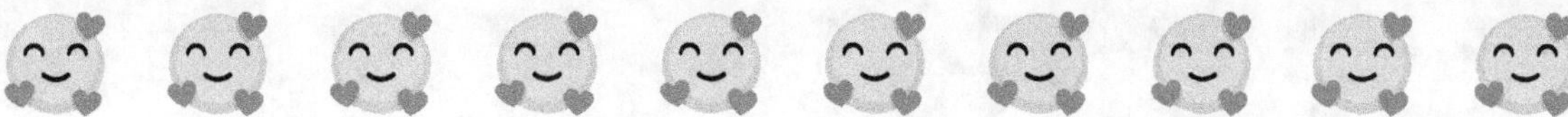

12. Lentil Soup with Vegetables

Let's do that and fill in the time here

 Prep Time :   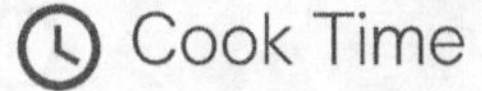 Cook Time :   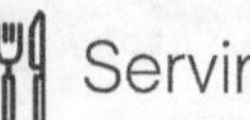 Servings :

Write 5 friends with whom you want to share this dish

....
....
....
....
....

Is this dish easy or difficult for you to make?

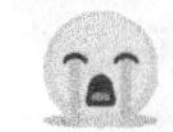 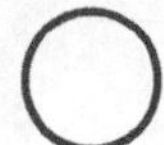 ○   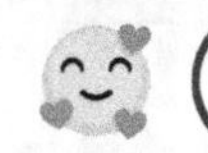 ○

INGREDIENTS

- 1 tbsp olive oil
- 1 onion, diced
- 3 cloves garlic, minced
- 2 carrots, peeled and diced
- 2 celery stalks, diced
- 1 cup dried brown or green lentils, rinsed
- 4 cups low-sodium vegetable or chicken broth
- 1 (14.5 oz) can diced tomatoes
- 2 cups chopped kale or spinach
- 1 tsp dried thyme
- 1 tsp dried oregano
- Salt and pepper to taste

1. In a large pot or Dutch oven, heat the olive oil over medium heat.

2. Add the diced onion and sauté for 3-4 minutes, until translucent.

3. Add the minced garlic and sauté for an additional minute, until fragrant.

4. Stir in the diced carrots and celery, and cook for 5-7 minutes, until slightly softened.

5. Add the rinsed lentils, vegetable or chicken broth, and diced tomatoes. Bring the mixture to a boil.

6. Reduce the heat to low, cover the pot, and simmer for 20-25 minutes, or until the lentils are tender.

7. Stir in the chopped kale or spinach, dried thyme, and dried oregano. Cook for an additional 5 minutes, until the greens are wilted.

8. Season the soup with salt and pepper to taste. Serve the lentil soup hot, garnished with additional chopped herbs or a drizzle of olive oil, if desired.

This lentil soup is a great option for a menopausal diet for several reasons:

1. Lentils are an excellent source of plant-based protein, fiber, and complex carbohydrates, which can help support sustained energy and feelings of fullness during menopause.
2. The vegetables, such as carrots, celery, and greens, provide a variety of vitamins, minerals, and antioxidants that can support overall health during menopause

How would you rate this dish?

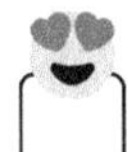 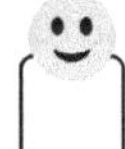 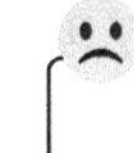 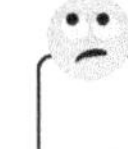 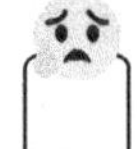

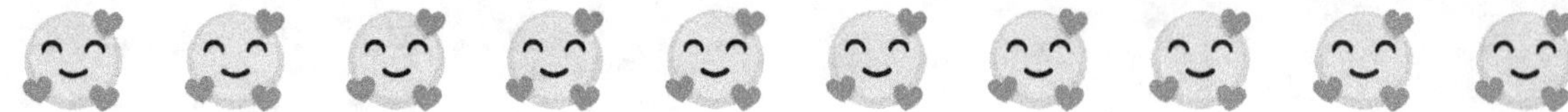

13. Quinoa Salad with Chickpeas, Cucumbers, and Tomatoes

 *Let's do that and fill in the time here* Prep Time :   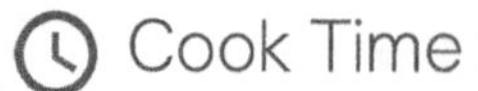 Cook Time :   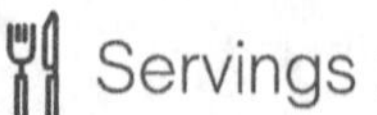 Servings :

Write 5 friends with whom you want to share this dish

....

....

....

....

....

Is this dish easy or difficult for you to make?

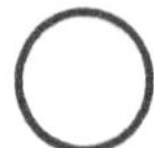 ◯    ◯

INGREDIENTS

- 1 cup cooked quinoa, cooled
- 1 (15 oz) can chickpeas, rinsed and drained
- 1 cup diced cucumber
- 1 cup cherry or grape tomatoes, halved
- 1/4 cup chopped fresh parsley
- 2 tbsp olive oil
- 2 tbsp lemon juice
- 1 tsp Dijon mustard
- 1 garlic clove, minced
- Salt and pepper to taste

1. In a large bowl, combine the cooked quinoa, chickpeas, diced cucumber, halved tomatoes, and chopped parsley.

2. In a small bowl, whisk together the olive oil, lemon juice, Dijon mustard, and minced garlic. Season with salt and pepper to taste.

3. Pour the dressing over the quinoa salad and toss gently to coat.

4. Refrigerate the salad for at least 30 minutes to allow the flavors to meld. Serve chilled or at room temperature.

This quinoa salad is a great option for a menopausal diet for several reasons:

1. Quinoa is a nutrient-dense whole grain that provides complex carbohydrates, protein, and fiber, which can help support sustained energy and feelings of fullness during menopause.

2. Chickpeas are a good source of plant-based protein, fiber, and complex carbohydrates, which can help maintain muscle mass and support overall health.

3. Cucumbers and tomatoes are hydrating and provide a variety of vitamins, minerals, and antioxidants that can support overall health during menopause.

4. The olive oil and lemon juice in the dressing provide healthy fats and vitamin C, which can help reduce inflammation and potentially alleviate some menopausal symptoms

How would you rate this dish?

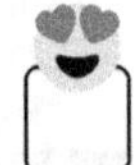 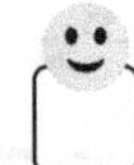  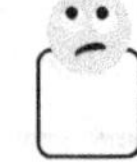 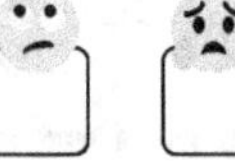 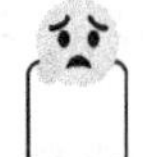

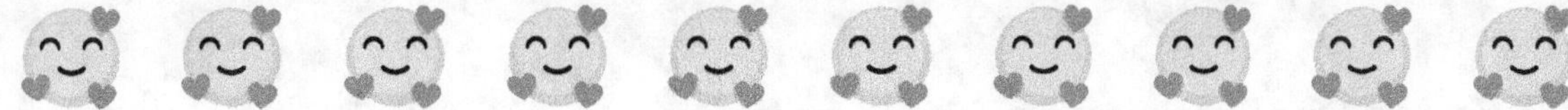

14. Whole Grain Wrap with Turkey, Hummus, and Veggies

 Prep Time : 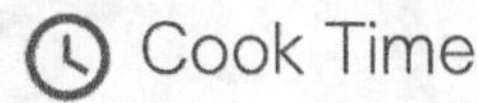 Cook Time : 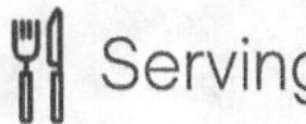 Servings :

Is this dish easy or difficult for you to make?

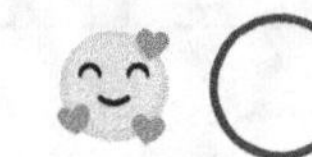

Write 5 friends with whom you want to share this dish

INGREDIENTS

- 1 whole grain tortilla or wrap
- 2-3 tbsp hummus
- 3 oz sliced turkey breast
- 1/2 cup mixed greens (such as spinach, arugula, or kale)
- 1/4 cup sliced cucumber
- 1/4 cup sliced bell pepper
- 1 tbsp crumbled feta cheese (optional)

1. Spread the hummus evenly over the whole grain tortilla or wrap.

2. Layer the sliced turkey breast over the hummus.

3. Top the turkey with the mixed greens, sliced cucumber, and sliced bell pepper.

4. If desired, sprinkle the crumbled feta cheese over the vegetables.

5. Carefully roll up the wrap, tucking in the sides as you go. Slice the wrap in half diagonally and serve immediately.

This whole grain wrap is a great option for a menopausal diet for several reasons:

1. Whole grain tortillas or wraps provide complex carbohydrates, fiber, and nutrients that can help support sustained energy and overall health during menopause.
2. Turkey is a lean source of protein, which can help maintain muscle mass and support bone health.
3. Hummus is a good source of plant-based protein, fiber, and healthy fats, which can help promote feelings of fullness.
4. The mixed greens, cucumber, and bell pepper provide a variety of vitamins, minerals, and antioxidants that can support overall health during menopause.
5. The optional feta cheese adds a boost of calcium, which is important for maintaining bone health during menopause.

How would you rate this dish?

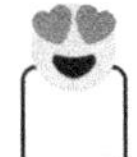   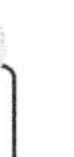 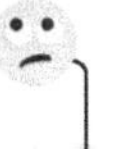 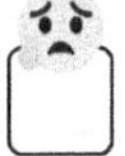

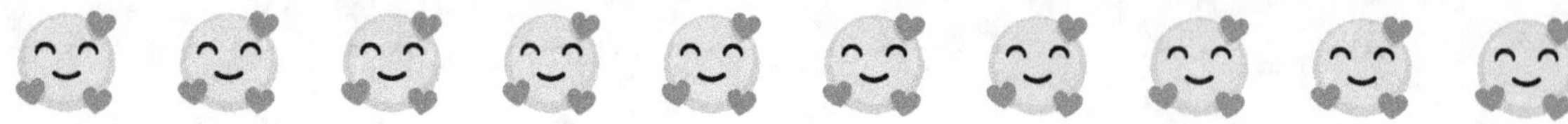

15. Spinach and Strawberry Salad with Poppy Seed Dressing

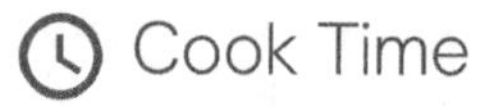 Prep Time :   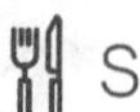 Cook Time :   Servings :

Write 5 friends with whom you want to share this dish

....

....

....

....

....

Is this dish easy or difficult for you to make?

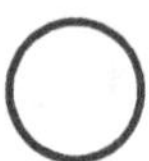 ◯   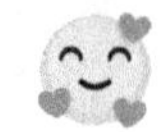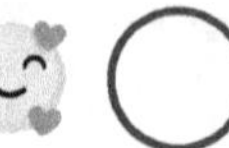 ◯

INGREDIENTS

Salad:
- 5 cups fresh spinach leaves
- 1 cup fresh strawberries, sliced
- 1/4 cup sliced almonds
- 2 tbsp crumbled feta cheese (optional)

Poppy Seed Dressing:
- 2 tbsp olive oil
- 2 tbsp white wine vinegar
- 1 tbsp honey
- 1 tsp Dijon mustard
- 1 tsp poppy seeds
- Salt and pepper to taste

1. In a large salad bowl, combine the fresh spinach leaves, sliced strawberries, sliced almonds, and crumbled feta cheese (if using).
2. In a small bowl, whisk together the olive oil, white wine vinegar, honey, Dijon mustard, and poppy seeds to make the dressing. Season with salt and pepper to taste.
3. Drizzle the poppy seed dressing over the salad and toss gently to coat.
4. Serve the spinach and strawberry salad immediately.

This spinach and strawberry salad is a great option for a menopausal diet for several reasons:

1. Spinach is a nutrient-dense leafy green that provides a variety of vitamins, minerals, and antioxidants that can support overall health during menopause.
2. Strawberries are a good source of vitamin C, which can help support immune function and potentially alleviate some menopausal symptoms.
3. Almonds are a rich source of healthy fats, protein, and fiber, which can help promote feelings of fullness and support bone health.
4. The poppy seed dressing is made with healthy fats from olive oil, as well as a touch of honey for sweetness, without the need for added sugars.
5. The salad is low in calories and high in nutrients, making it a balanced and satisfying option for a menopausal diet.

This colorful and flavorful salad can be a great addition to your menopausal meal plan.

How would you rate this dish?

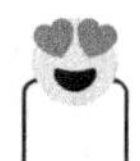 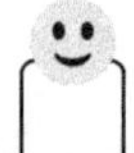 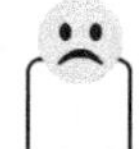 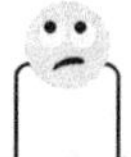 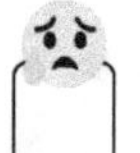

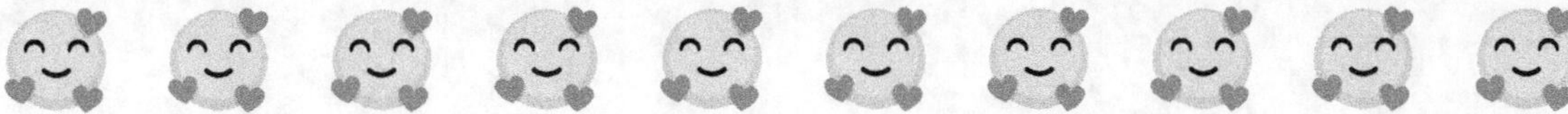

16. Brown Rice Bowl with Black Beans, Corn, and Salsa

Let's do that and fill in the time here

 Prep Time :

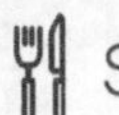 Cook Time :

Servings :

Write 5 friends with whom you want to share this dish

....

....

....

....

....

INGREDIENTS

- 1 cup cooked brown rice
- 1 (15 oz) can black beans, rinsed and drained
- 1 cup frozen corn, thawed
- 1/2 cup fresh salsa
- 1 avocado, diced
- 2 tbsp crumbled feta cheese (optional)
- Lime wedges for serving

Is this dish easy or difficult for you to make?

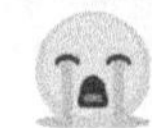 ◯

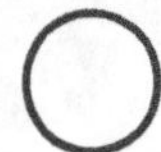 ◯

1. In a medium bowl, combine the cooked brown rice, rinsed and drained black beans, and thawed corn.

2. Top the rice and bean mixture with the fresh salsa, diced avocado, and crumbled feta cheese (if using).

3. Serve the brown rice bowl with lime wedges on the side.

This brown rice bowl is a great option for a menopausal diet for several reasons:

1. Brown rice is a whole grain that provides complex carbohydrates, fiber, and nutrients that can help support sustained energy and overall health during menopause.
2. Black beans are a good source of plant-based protein, fiber, and complex carbohydrates, which can help maintain muscle mass and support feelings of fullness.
3. Corn provides a source of complex carbohydrates, as well as vitamins and minerals that can support overall health.
4. Fresh salsa is a flavorful way to add vegetables, vitamins, and antioxidants to the dish without the need for excessive sodium or added sugars.
5. Avocado is a rich source of healthy monounsaturated fats, which can help promote feelings of fullness and support heart health.
6. The optional feta cheese adds a boost of calcium, which is important for maintaining bone health during menopause.

This colorful and balanced meal can be a great option for a quick and nutritious lunch or dinner as part of a menopausal diet.

How would you rate this dish?

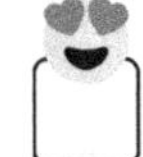 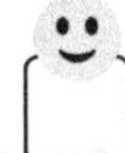  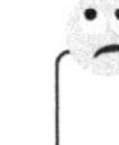 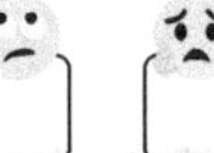

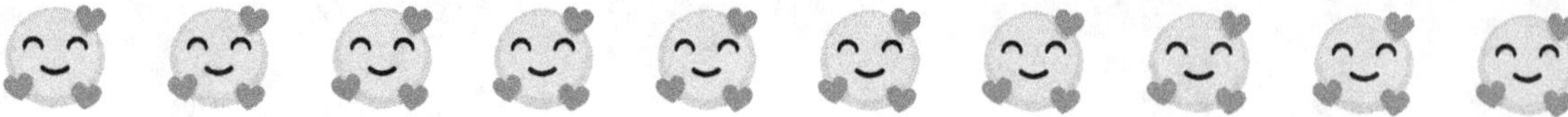

17. Roasted Beet Salad with Goat Cheese and Walnuts

Let's do that and fill in the time here

 Prep Time :

Cook Time :

Servings :

Is this dish easy or difficult for you to make?

 ◯   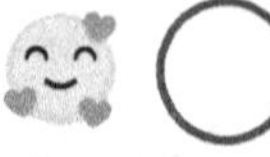 ◯

Write 5 friends with whom you want to share this dish

INGREDIENTS

- 3 medium-sized beets, peeled and cut into 1-inch cubes
- 1 tbsp olive oil
- Salt and pepper to taste
- 4 cups mixed greens (such as spinach, arugula, or kale)
- 2 oz crumbled goat cheese
- 1/4 cup chopped walnuts
- 2 tbsp balsamic vinegar
- 1 tsp Dijon mustard
- 1 tbsp honey (optional)

1. Preheat your oven to 400°F (200°C).
2. Toss the cubed beets with the olive oil, salt, and pepper. Spread them out on a baking sheet and roast for 25-30 minutes, or until the beets are tender and lightly caramelized.
3. In a large salad bowl, combine the roasted beets, mixed greens, crumbled goat cheese, and chopped walnuts.
4. In a small bowl, whisk together the balsamic vinegar, Dijon mustard, and honey (if using) to make the dressing.
5. Drizzle the dressing over the salad and toss gently to coat.
6. Serve the roasted beet salad immediately.

This roasted beet salad is a great option for a menopausal diet for several reasons:

1. Beets are a good source of folate, which can help support red blood cell production and potentially alleviate some menopausal symptoms.
2. Greens like spinach and arugula are nutrient-dense and provide a variety of vitamins, minerals, and antioxidants that can support overall health during menopause.
3. Goat cheese is a good source of protein and calcium, which can help maintain bone health.
4. Walnuts are a rich source of omega-3 fatty acids, which can have anti-inflammatory properties and potentially alleviate some menopausal symptoms.
5. The balsamic vinegar and Dijon mustard in the dressing provide a flavorful way to add healthy fats and reduce the need for added sugars.

How would you rate this dish?

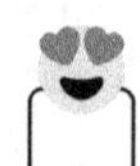 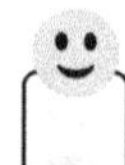 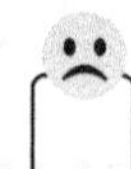 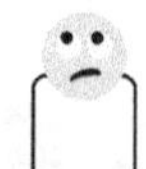 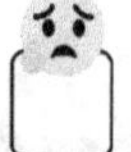

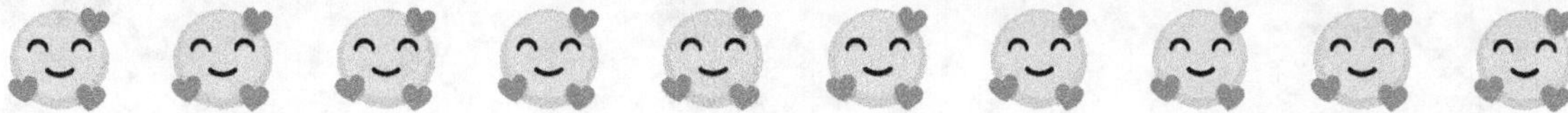

18. Stuffed Bell Peppers with Quinoa and Black Beans

 Prep Time :

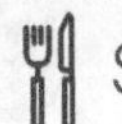 Cook Time :

Servings :

Write 5 friends with whom you want to share this dish

....

....

....

....

....

Is this dish easy or difficult for you to make?

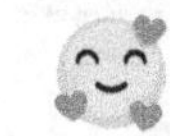 ○   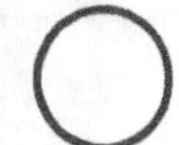 ○

INGREDIENTS

- 4 bell peppers (any color), halved lengthwise and seeds removed
- 1 cup cooked quinoa
- 1 (15 oz) can black beans, rinsed and drained
- 1 cup diced tomatoes
- 1/2 cup shredded cheddar or Monterey Jack cheese
- 2 tbsp chopped fresh cilantro
- 1 tsp ground cumin
- Salt and pepper to taste

1. Preheat your oven to 375°F (190°C).
2. Arrange the bell pepper halves in a baking dish or on a rimmed baking sheet.
3. In a medium bowl, combine the cooked quinoa, black beans, diced tomatoes, shredded cheese, chopped cilantro, and ground cumin. Season with salt and pepper to taste.
4. Spoon the quinoa and black bean mixture evenly into the bell pepper halves.
5. Bake the stuffed bell peppers for 25-30 minutes, or until the peppers are tender and the filling is heated through.
6. Serve the stuffed bell peppers warm.

This stuffed bell pepper dish is a great option for a menopausal diet for several reasons:

1. Bell peppers are a good source of vitamins, minerals, and antioxidants that can support overall health during menopause.
2. Quinoa is a nutrient-dense whole grain that provides complex carbohydrates, protein, and fiber, which can help support sustained energy and feelings of fullness.
3. Black beans are a good source of plant-based protein, fiber, and complex carbohydrates, which can help maintain muscle mass and support feelings of fullness.
4. The shredded cheese provides a boost of calcium, which is important for maintaining bone health during menopause.
5. The dish is relatively low in added sugars and high in nutrients, making it a balanced and satisfying option for a menopausal diet.

How would you rate this dish?

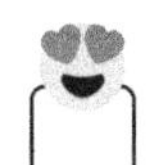 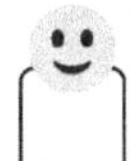 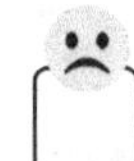 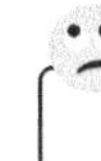 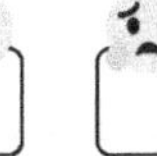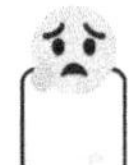

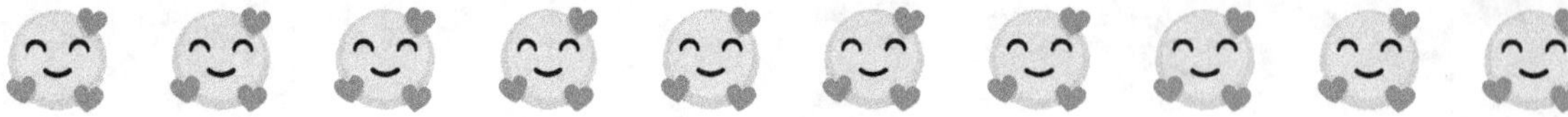

19. Greek Salad with Feta Cheese and Kalamata Olives

 *Let's do that and fill in the time here* 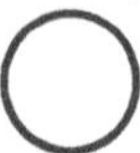 Prep Time : 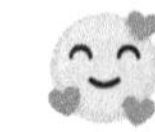 Cook Time : 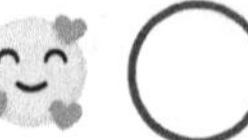 Servings :

Write 5 friends with whom you want to share this dish

Is this dish easy or difficult for you to make?
 ○   ○

INGREDIENTS

- 5 cups mixed greens (such as romaine, spinach, or arugula)
- 1 cup cherry tomatoes, halved
- 1/2 cucumber, sliced
- 1/4 red onion, thinly sliced
- 1/4 cup crumbled feta cheese
- 1/4 cup Kalamata olives, pitted and halved
- 2 tbsp olive oil
- 1 tbsp red wine vinegar
- 1 tsp dried oregano
- Salt and pepper to taste

1. In a large salad bowl, combine the mixed greens, cherry tomatoes, sliced cucumber, and thinly sliced red onion.
2. Sprinkle the crumbled feta cheese and halved Kalamata olives over the top of the salad.
3. In a small bowl, whisk together the olive oil, red wine vinegar, and dried oregano to make the dressing.
4. Drizzle the dressing over the salad and toss gently to coat.
5. Season the salad with salt and pepper to taste.
6. Serve the Greek salad immediately.

This Greek salad is a great option for a menopausal diet for several reasons:

1. The mixed greens, tomatoes, and cucumber provide a variety of vitamins, minerals, and antioxidants that can support overall health during menopause.
2. Feta cheese is a good source of calcium, which is important for maintaining bone health.
3. Kalamata olives are a source of healthy monounsaturated fats, which can help promote feelings of fullness and support heart health.
4. The olive oil and red wine vinegar in the dressing provide additional healthy fats and a flavorful way to dress the salad without the need for excessive sodium or added sugars.
5. The salad is relatively low in calories and high in nutrients, making it a balanced and satisfying option for a menopausal diet.

This colorful and refreshing salad can be a great addition to your menopausal meal plan.

How would you rate this dish?

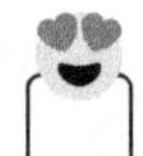 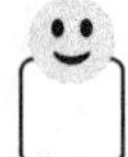 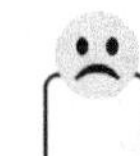 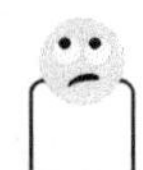 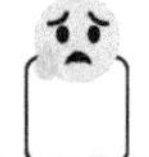

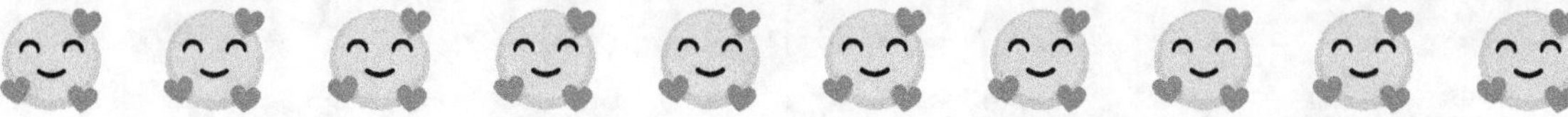

20. Zucchini Noodles with Pesto and Cherry Tomatoes

 Prep Time : 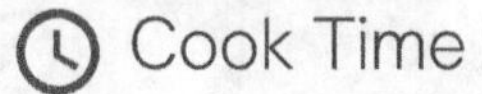 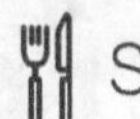 Cook Time : Servings :

Is this dish easy or difficult for you to make?

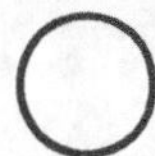 ◯ 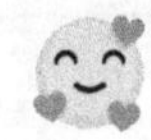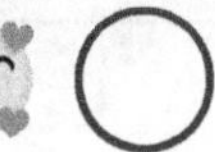 ◯

Write 5 friends with whom you want to share this dish

INGREDIENTS

- 2 medium zucchini, spiralized or julienned into noodles
- 1/2 cup homemade or store-bought basil pesto
- 1 cup cherry tomatoes, halved
- 2 tbsp toasted pine nuts (optional)
- 2 tbsp grated Parmesan cheese (optional)
- Salt and pepper to taste

1. In a large bowl, combine the spiralized or julienned zucchini noodles with the basil pesto, making sure the noodles are evenly coated.
2. Gently fold in the halved cherry tomatoes.
3. Top the zucchini noodle mixture with the toasted pine nuts (if using) and grated Parmesan cheese (if using).
4. Season with salt and pepper to taste.
5. Serve the zucchini noodles with pesto and cherry tomatoes immediately.

This zucchini noodle dish is a great option for a menopausal diet for several reasons:

1. Zucchini is a low-calorie, nutrient-dense vegetable that provides a good source of vitamins, minerals, and antioxidants to support overall health during menopause.
2. Basil pesto is a flavorful way to add healthy fats from the olive oil and pine nuts, as well as vitamins and antioxidants from the fresh basil.
3. Cherry tomatoes are a good source of lycopene, an antioxidant that may help reduce the risk of certain health conditions associated with menopause.
4. The optional pine nuts and Parmesan cheese provide a boost of healthy fats and calcium, respectively, which can help support bone health during menopause.
5. The dish is low in carbohydrates and high in nutrients, making it a balanced and satisfying option for a menopausal diet.

This light and refreshing zucchini noodle dish can be a great addition to your menopausal meal plan.

How would you rate this dish?

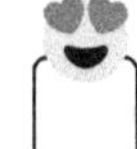 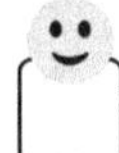  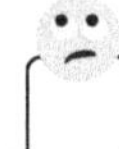 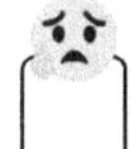

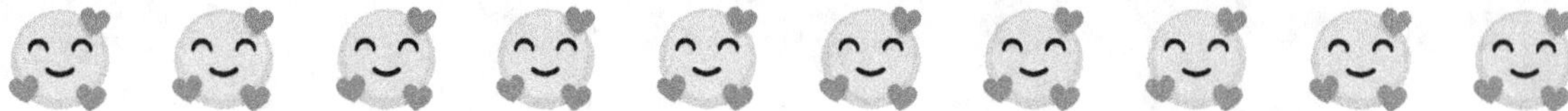

21. Apple Slices with Almond Butter

 *Let's do that and fill in the time here*

Prep Time :   Cook Time :   Servings :

Write 5 friends with whom you want to share this dish
....
....
....
....
....

Is this dish easy or difficult for you to make?

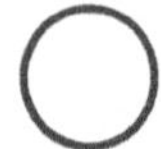 ◯   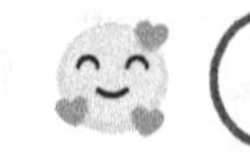 ◯

INGREDIENTS

- 1 medium-sized apple, cored and sliced
- 2 tbsp natural almond butter

1. Wash and slice the apple into thin wedges or slices.

2. Spread a small amount of almond butter (about 1-2 tsp) onto each apple slice.

That's it! This snack is ready to enjoy.

This apple and almond butter combination is a great option for a menopausal diet for several reasons:

1. Apples are a good source of fiber, vitamins, and antioxidants, which can help support overall health during menopause.

2. Almond butter is a rich source of healthy monounsaturated fats, protein, and fiber, which can help promote feelings of fullness and support heart health.

3. The combination of the crisp apple and creamy almond butter provides a satisfying and balanced snack.

4. This snack is low in added sugars and high in nutrients, making it a healthier option compared to many processed snacks.

This simple and portable snack can be a great way to incorporate more nutrient-dense foods into your menopausal diet. The healthy fats and fiber from the almond butter and apple can help keep you feeling full and satisfied between meals. Let me know if you have any other questions!

How would you rate this dish?

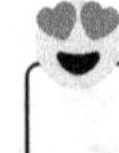 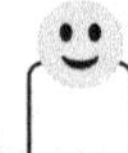 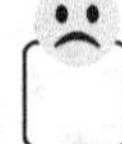 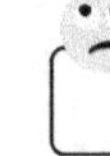 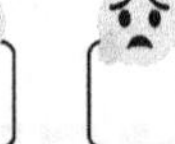

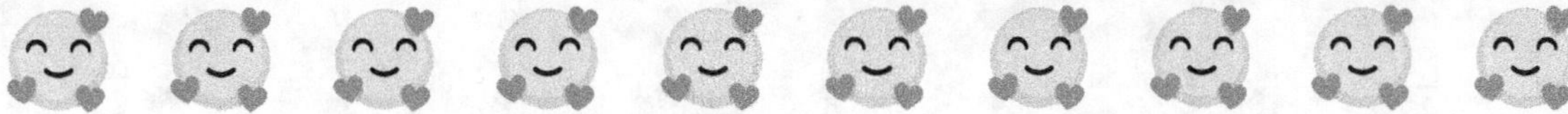

22. Hummus with Carrot and Celery Sticks

 Prep Time :   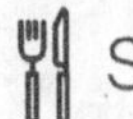 Cook Time :   Servings :

Is this dish easy or difficult for you to make?

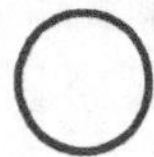 ◯   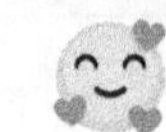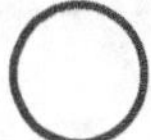 ◯

Write 5 friends with whom you want to share this dish

....

....

....

....

....

INGREDIENTS

- 1 (15 oz) can chickpeas/garbanzo beans, drained and rinsed
- 2 tbsp tahini (sesame seed paste)
- 2 tbsp fresh lemon juice
- 1 garlic clove, minced
- 2 tbsp olive oil
- 1/4 tsp ground cumin
- Salt and pepper to taste
- 1 cup baby carrots, washed and trimmed
- 1 cup celery sticks, washed and trimmed

1. In a food processor, combine the chickpeas, tahini, lemon juice, garlic, olive oil, and cumin. Process until smooth and creamy, scraping down the sides as needed.

2. Season the hummus with salt and pepper to taste. Transfer to a serving bowl.

3. Arrange the carrot and celery sticks around the hummus in the serving bowl.

4. Serve immediately with the carrot and celery sticks for dipping.

Enjoy this healthy and flavorful hummus dip with the fresh crunchy vegetables! The combination of the creamy hummus and the crisp carrots and celery makes for a delicious and nutritious snack or appetizer.

How would you rate this dish?

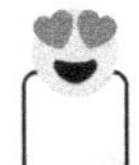 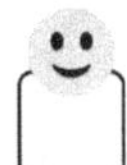 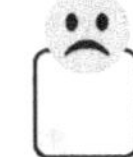 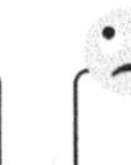 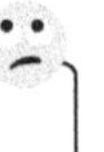 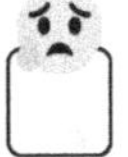

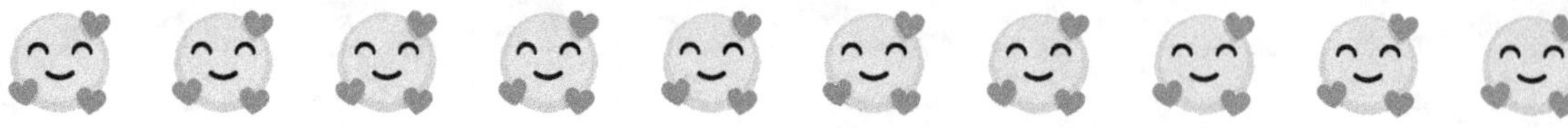

23. Mixed Nuts and Seeds

 Prep Time : 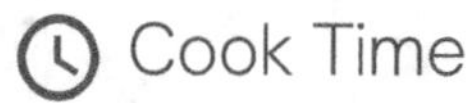 Cook Time : 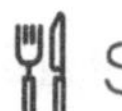 Servings :

Is this dish easy or difficult for you to make?

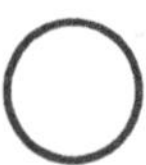 ◯ 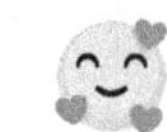 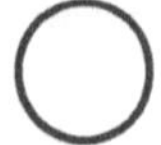 ◯

Write 5 friends with whom you want to share this dish

....

....

....

....

....

INGREDIENTS

- 1/2 cup raw almonds
- 1/2 cup raw walnuts
- 1/4 cup raw pumpkin seeds
- 1/4 cup raw sunflower seeds
- 2 tbsp chia seeds
- 1 tbsp ground flaxseeds
- 1 tsp ground cinnamon (optional)
- 1/4 tsp sea salt (optional)

1. In a medium bowl, combine the almonds, walnuts, pumpkin seeds, sunflower seeds, chia seeds, and ground flaxseeds.

2. If desired, sprinkle the cinnamon and sea salt over the nut and seed mixture and stir to coat evenly.

3. Transfer the mixed nuts and seeds to an airtight container or resealable bag. Store at room temperature for up to 2 weeks.

Why this is a great menopause diet snack:

- Nuts and seeds are rich in healthy fats, protein, fiber, and a variety of vitamins and minerals that can help support women's health during menopause.

- Almonds and walnuts contain phytoestrogens that can help balance hormone levels.

- Pumpkin seeds are a good source of magnesium, which can help relieve menopause symptoms like hot flashes and mood swings.

- Chia and flaxseeds are high in omega-3 fatty acids, which have anti-inflammatory properties.

- The cinnamon adds a touch of sweetness and may help regulate blood sugar levels.

This versatile mixed nuts and seeds snack can be enjoyed on its own, sprinkled on yogurt or oatmeal, or used as a topping for salads. It's a nutritious and satisfying option for women going through menopause.

How would you rate this dish?

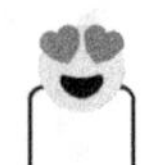 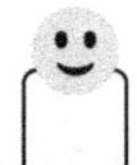 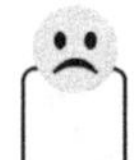 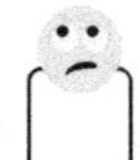 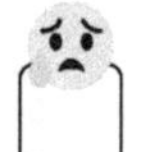

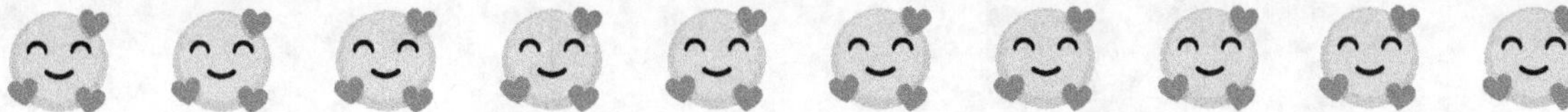

24. Edamame with Sea Salt

 Prep Time :   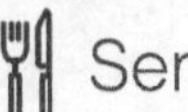 Cook Time :   Servings :

Is this dish easy or difficult for you to make?

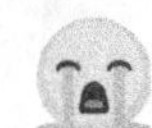 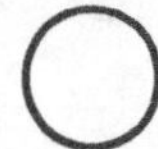 ◯   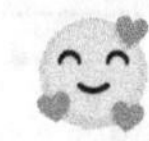 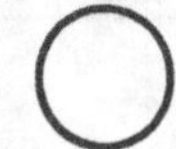 ◯

Write 5 friends with whom you want to share this dish

....

....

....

....

....

INGREDIENTS

- 1 cup frozen edamame, in the pod
- 1/4 tsp sea salt

1. Bring a medium pot of water to a boil.

2. Add the frozen edamame pods to the boiling water and cook for 5-7 minutes, or until the pods are tender.

3. Drain the edamame and transfer them to a serving bowl.

4. Sprinkle the sea salt over the edamame and toss gently to coat.

5. Serve the edamame with sea salt warm or at room temperature.

This edamame with sea salt snack is a great option for a menopausal diet for several reasons:

1. Edamame is a good source of plant-based protein, fiber, and nutrients that can help support overall health during menopause.
2. The protein and fiber in edamame can help promote feelings of fullness and support sustained energy levels.
3. Sea salt is a minimally processed alternative to table salt, providing a flavorful way to season the edamame without the need for excessive sodium.
4. Edamame is a low-calorie, nutrient-dense snack that can be easily incorporated into a balanced menopausal diet.

This simple and satisfying snack can be a great way to incorporate more plant-based protein and fiber into your menopausal diet. The combination of the tender edamame pods and the crunchy sea salt makes for a delicious and nutritious treat.

How would you rate this dish?

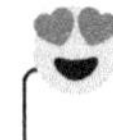 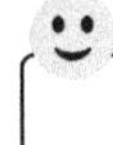 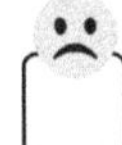 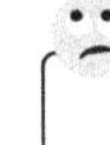 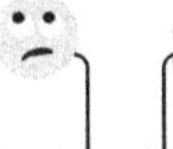 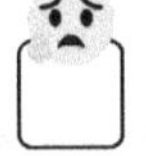

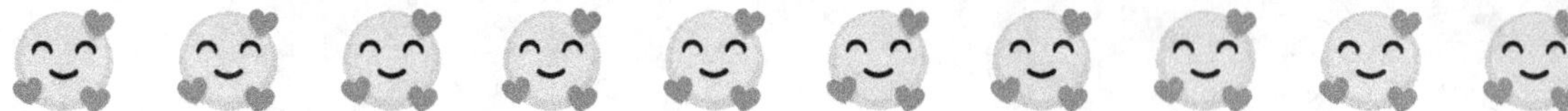

25. Fresh Berries with Greek Yogurt

 Prep Time :

 Cook Time :

Servings :

Write 5 friends with whom you want to share this dish

....

....

....

....

....

Is this dish easy or difficult for you to make?

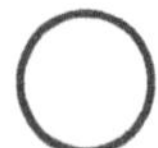 ◯   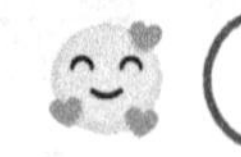 ◯

INGREDIENTS

- 1 cup mixed fresh berries (such as blueberries, raspberries, and/or strawberries)
- 1 cup plain Greek yogurt
- 1 tbsp honey (optional)
- 1 tbsp chopped walnuts or sliced almonds (optional)

1. In a bowl, gently mix the fresh berries with the plain Greek yogurt.

2. If desired, drizzle the honey over the top of the berry and yogurt mixture.

3. Sprinkle the chopped walnuts or sliced almonds over the top (if using).

4. Serve immediately or refrigerate until ready to enjoy.

This fresh berries with Greek yogurt dish is a great option for a menopausal diet for several reasons:

1. Berries are rich in antioxidants, fiber, and vitamins that can help support overall health and potentially alleviate some menopausal symptoms.
2. Greek yogurt is an excellent source of protein, which can help maintain muscle mass and support bone health during menopause.
3. The optional honey provides a touch of sweetness without using refined sugar, which can be helpful for managing blood sugar levels.
4. The nuts, such as walnuts or almonds, add a boost of healthy fats, protein, and fiber, which can help promote feelings of fullness and support bone health.

This simple and versatile dish can be enjoyed as a snack, breakfast, or light dessert as part of a balanced menopausal diet. The combination of the fresh berries, protein-rich Greek yogurt, and optional honey and nuts makes for a nutritious and satisfying treat.

How would you rate this dish?

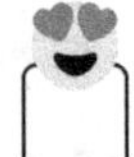 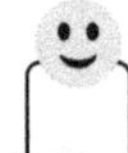 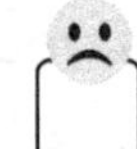 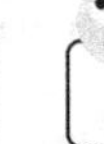 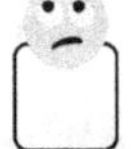 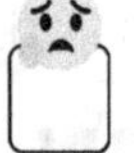

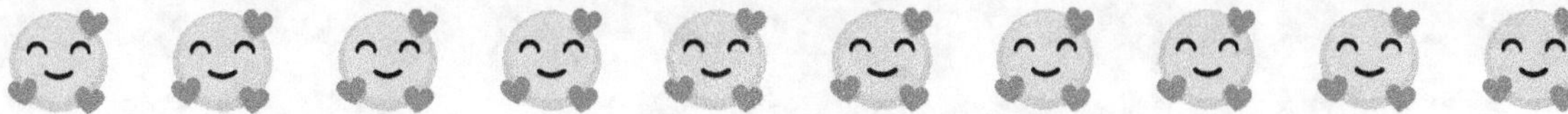

26. Sliced Bell Peppers with Guacamole

 Prep Time :

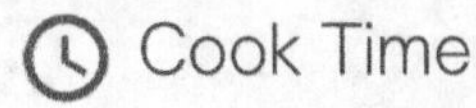 Cook Time :

 Servings :

Is this dish easy or difficult for you to make?

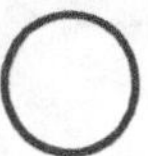 ◯   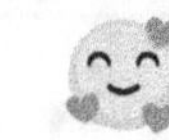 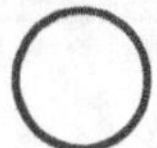 ◯

Write 5 friends with whom you want to share this dish

....

....

....

....

....

INGREDIENTS

For the Guacamole:
- 2 ripe avocados, pitted and diced
- 1 tablespoon fresh lime juice
- 2 tablespoons finely chopped red onion
- 1 garlic clove, minced
- 2 tablespoons chopped fresh cilantro (optional)
- 1/4 teaspoon sea salt
- 1/4 teaspoon ground cumin

For the Bell Peppers:
- 2 bell peppers (any color), washed and sliced into strips

1. In a medium bowl, mash the avocado chunks with a fork or potato masher until slightly chunky.

2. Add the lime juice, onion, garlic, cilantro (if using), salt, and cumin. Stir to combine.

3. Taste and adjust seasoning as needed.

4. Arrange the bell pepper strips on a serving platter or plate.

5. Scoop the guacamole into a small bowl and place it in the center of the plate with the bell pepper strips around it.

Why this is a great menopause diet snack:

- Bell peppers are an excellent source of vitamin C, which can help support the immune system during menopause.
- The capsaicin in bell peppers may help alleviate hot flashes and night sweats.
- Avocados are rich in healthy monounsaturated fats, which can help maintain healthy cholesterol levels and support heart health.
- Avocados also contain phytoestrogens, which can help balance hormone levels during menopause.
- The combination of the crunchy bell peppers and the creamy, flavorful guacamole provides a satisfying and nutritious snack.

This Sliced Bell Peppers with Guacamole dish is a great way to incorporate nutrient-dense, menopause-friendly ingredients into your diet. Enjoy it as a healthy snack or appetizer.

How would you rate this dish?

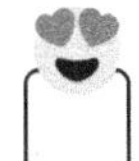 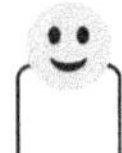  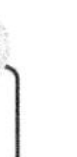 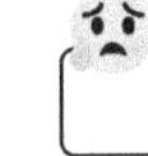

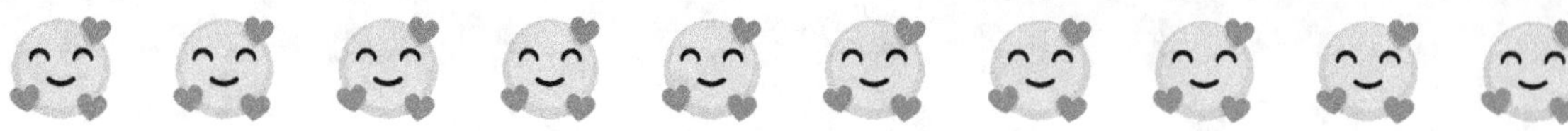

27. Kale Chips

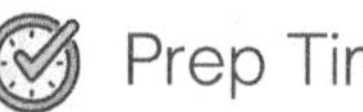 Prep Time :    Cook Time :   Servings :

Write 5 friends with whom you want to share this dish

....

....

....

....

....

Is this dish easy or difficult for you to make?

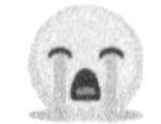 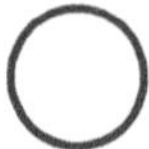 ◯   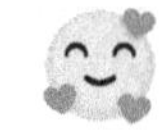 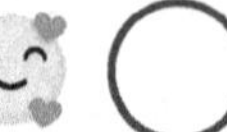 ◯

INGREDIENTS

- 1 bunch kale, washed and dried thoroughly
- 1-2 tbsp olive oil
- 1/2 tsp sea salt (or to taste)
- Optional seasonings: garlic powder, onion powder, paprika, cayenne pepper, etc.

1. Preheat your oven to 325°F (165°C).

2. Wash the kale and pat it completely dry with paper towels or a clean kitchen towel. This is important to ensure the kale chips get crispy.

3. Tear or cut the kale leaves into bite-sized pieces, discarding any tough stems.

4. Place the kale pieces in a large bowl and drizzle with the olive oil. Use your hands to massage the oil into the kale, making sure all the leaves are evenly coated.

5. Sprinkle the sea salt (and any other desired seasonings) over the kale and toss to distribute evenly.

6. Arrange the kale pieces in a single layer on baking sheets lined with parchment paper or a silicone baking mat.

7. Bake for 12-15 minutes, flipping the kale halfway through, until the leaves are crispy and lightly browned.

8. Remove the kale chips from the oven and let them cool completely before serving.

Enjoy these homemade kale chips as a healthy, flavorful alternative to traditional potato chips or other salty snacks.

How would you rate this dish?

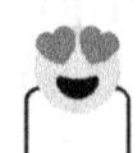 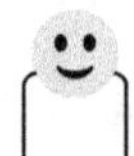 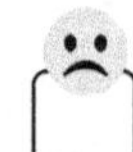 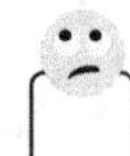 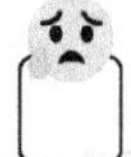

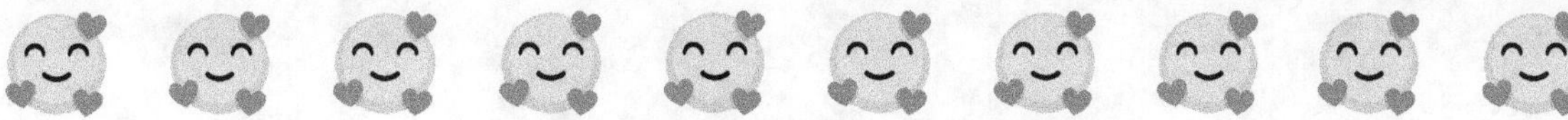

28. Hard-Boiled Eggs

 Prep Time : 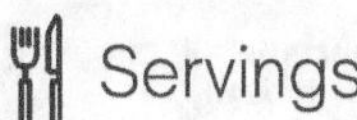 Cook Time : Servings :

Let's do that and fill in the time here

Is this dish easy or difficult for you to make?

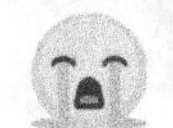 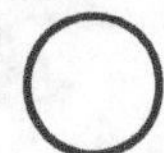 ◯ 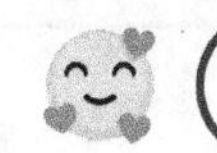 ◯

Write 5 friends with whom you want to share this dish

....

....

....

....

....

INGREDIENTS

- 6 large eggs

1. Place the eggs in a single layer in a saucepan and cover with cold water by 1 inch.

2. Bring the water to a boil over high heat. Once the water reaches a full boil, remove the pan from the heat and cover.

3. Let the eggs sit in the hot water for the following times:
- Soft-boiled: 6-7 minutes
- Hard-boiled: 12 minutes

4. Drain the hot water and cover the eggs with cold water. Let sit for 5 minutes.

5. Gently tap the eggs against the counter to crack the shells, then peel starting from the wider end of the egg. Rinse the peeled eggs under cold water to remove any remaining shell fragments.

Why hard-boiled eggs are great for a menopause diet:

- Eggs are an excellent source of high-quality protein, which can help maintain muscle mass and support overall health during menopause.

- The yolks are rich in choline, a nutrient that is important for brain health and may help alleviate cognitive changes associated with menopause.

- Eggs contain vitamin D, which is crucial for bone health and can help prevent osteoporosis, a common issue for menopausal women.

How would you rate this dish?

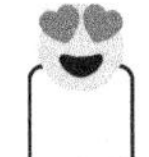 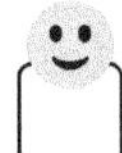  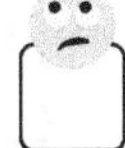 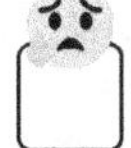

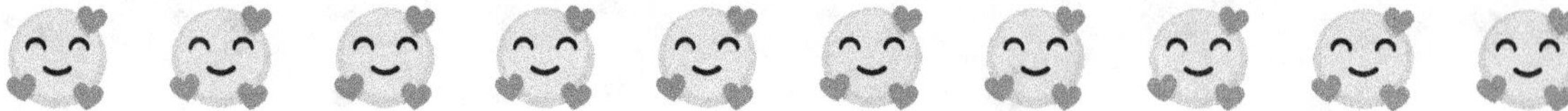

29. Whole Grain Crackers with Cheese

 Prep Time :   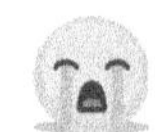 Cook Time :   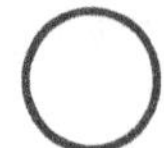 Servings :

Write 5 friends with whom you want to share this dish
....
....
....
....
....

Is this dish easy or difficult for you to make?

 ◯   🙂 ◯

INGREDIENTS

- 1 package (4-6 oz) whole grain crackers
- 2-3 oz low-fat or reduced-fat cheese (such as cheddar, gouda, or feta), sliced or crumbled

1. Arrange the whole grain crackers on a serving plate or platter.

2. Top each cracker with a slice or crumble of the cheese.

3. Serve immediately.

Why this is a great menopause diet snack:

- Whole grain crackers are a good source of complex carbohydrates, fiber, and B vitamins, which can help provide sustained energy and support overall health during menopause.

- The cheese provides high-quality protein, which is important for maintaining muscle mass and bone health as women go through menopause.

- Cheese is also a good source of calcium, which is crucial for preventing osteoporosis, a common issue for menopausal women.

- The combination of the whole grains and protein-rich cheese creates a satisfying and balanced snack that can help manage hunger and cravings.

- This snack is easy to prepare and can be customized with different types of whole grain crackers and cheeses to suit individual preferences.

Whole Grain Crackers with Cheese is a simple, nutritious, and versatile snack that can be a great addition to a menopause diet. It provides a good balance of carbohydrates, protein, and calcium to support women's health during this transition.

How would you rate this dish?

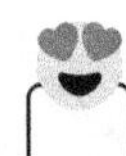 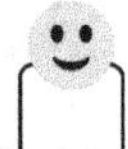 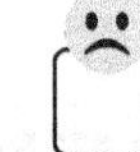 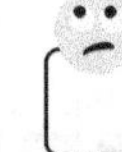 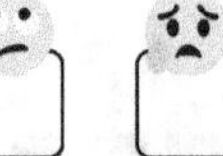 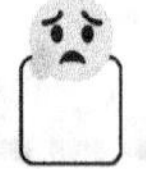

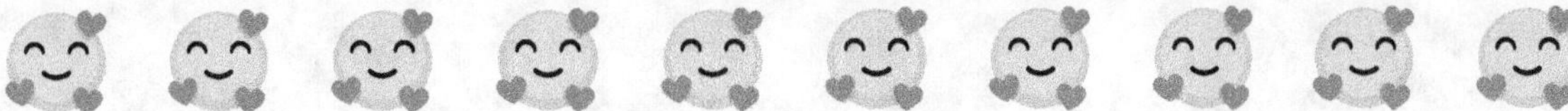

30. Smoothie with Spinach, Berries, and Chia Seeds

 Prep Time : 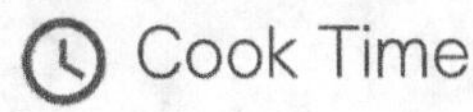 Cook Time :  Servings :

Is this dish easy or difficult for you to make?

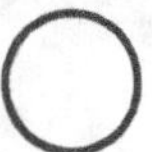 ○ 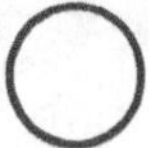 ○

Write 5 friends with whom you want to share this dish

INGREDIENTS

- 1 cup fresh spinach leaves
- 1 cup frozen mixed berries (such as blueberries, raspberries, and strawberries)
- 1 cup unsweetened almond milk (or milk of your choice)
- 1 tablespoon chia seeds
- 1 tablespoon honey or maple syrup (optional)
- 1/2 teaspoon vanilla extract (optional)

1. In a high-speed blender, combine the spinach, frozen berries, almond milk, chia seeds, honey/maple syrup (if using), and vanilla extract (if using).

2. Blend on high speed until the mixture is smooth and creamy, about 1-2 minutes. Pour the smoothie into a glass and enjoy immediately.

Why this is a great menopause diet smoothie:

- Spinach is a nutrient-dense leafy green that is rich in vitamins A, C, and K, as well as folate, which can help support overall health during menopause.

- Berries are packed with antioxidants, fiber, and phytoestrogens, which can help balance hormone levels and alleviate menopausal symptoms.

- Chia seeds are a great source of omega-3 fatty acids, fiber, and protein, all of which are important for menopausal women's health.

- Almond milk is a dairy-free, low-calorie option that provides calcium and other essential nutrients.

- The honey or maple syrup (if used) can add a touch of sweetness without the need for added sugars.

This Spinach, Berry, and Chia Seed Smoothie is a delicious and nutritious way to start your day or enjoy as a snack during menopause. The combination of leafy greens, antioxidant-rich berries, and nutrient-dense seeds makes it a well-balanced and menopause-friendly choice.

How would you rate this dish?

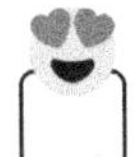 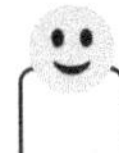  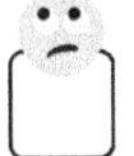 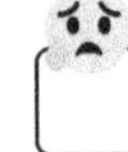

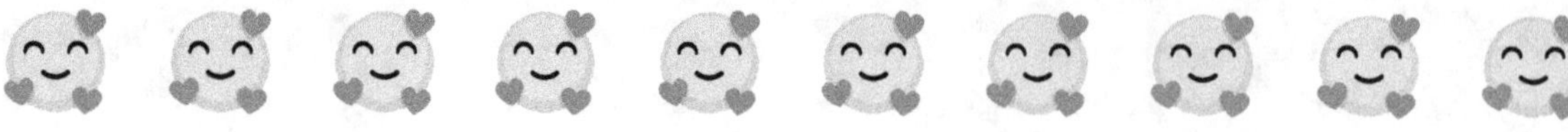

31. Grilled Salmon with Asparagus

 *Let's do that and fill in the time here*

 Prep Time :

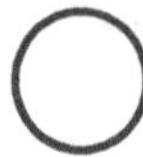 Cook Time :

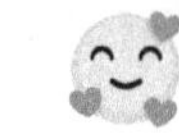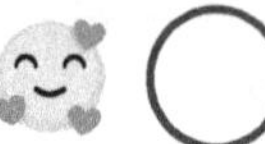 Servings :

Write 5 friends with whom you want to share this dish

....

....

....

....

....

Is this dish easy or difficult for you to make?

😭 ◯   🥰 ◯

INGREDIENTS

- 4 (6 oz) salmon fillets
- 1 lb asparagus, trimmed
- 2 tablespoons olive oil, divided
- 1 tablespoon lemon juice
- 2 garlic cloves, minced
- 1 teaspoon dried dill
- 1/2 teaspoon salt
- 1/4 teaspoon black pepper

1. Preheat your grill or grill pan to medium-high heat.

2. In a small bowl, whisk together 1 tablespoon of the olive oil, lemon juice, garlic, dill, salt, and pepper.

3. Place the salmon fillets and asparagus spears in a single layer on a large baking sheet or plate. Drizzle the remaining 1 tablespoon of olive oil over the asparagus and toss to coat.

4. Grill the salmon for 4-6 minutes per side, or until it flakes easily with a fork and reaches an internal temperature of 145°F (63°C).

5. Grill the asparagus for 5-7 minutes, turning occasionally, until tender-crisp.

6. Transfer the grilled salmon and asparagus to a serving platter. Drizzle the lemon-garlic-dill mixture over the top of the salmon.

7. Serve the Grilled Salmon with Asparagus immediately.

Enjoy this Grilled Salmon with Asparagus as a delicious and nutritious addition to your menopause diet.

How would you rate this dish?

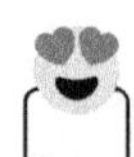 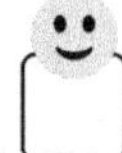 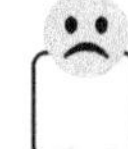 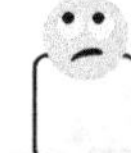 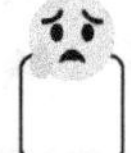

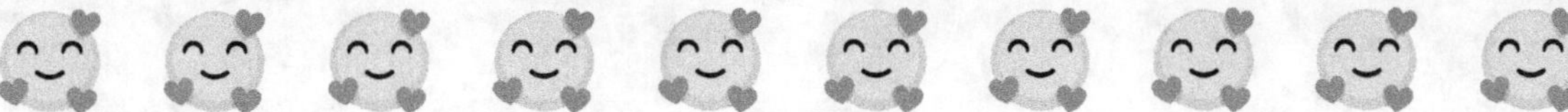

32. Chicken Stir-Fry with Broccoli and Bell Peppers

 *Let's do that and fill in the time here* 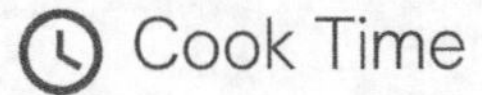 Prep Time : 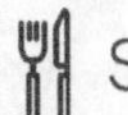 Cook Time : Servings :

Write 5 friends with whom you want to share this dish ....

Is this dish easy or difficult for you to make?

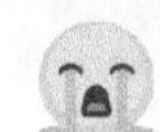 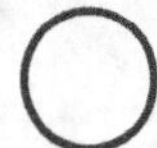 ◯    ◯

INGREDIENTS

- 1 lb boneless, skinless chicken breasts, cut into 1-inch pieces
- 2 tablespoons low-sodium soy sauce
- 1 tablespoon rice vinegar
- 1 teaspoon sesame oil
- 1 tablespoon cornstarch
- 2 tablespoons olive oil
- 3 cups broccoli florets
- 1 red bell pepper, sliced
- 1 yellow bell pepper, sliced
- 3 garlic cloves, minced
- 1 tablespoon grated fresh ginger
- 2 green onions, sliced (optional)
- Cooked brown rice, for serving

1. In a medium bowl, combine the chicken, soy sauce, rice vinegar, sesame oil, and cornstarch. Toss to coat the chicken and set aside.

2. Heat the olive oil in a large skillet or wok over high heat. Add the broccoli and bell peppers, and stir-fry for 3-4 minutes, until the vegetables are crisp-tender.

3. Add the garlic and ginger to the skillet and cook for 1 minute, stirring constantly, until fragrant.

4. Add the marinated chicken to the skillet and stir-fry for 5-7 minutes, or until the chicken is cooked through and no longer pink.

5. If desired, stir in the sliced green onions. Serve the chicken stir-fry immediately over cooked brown rice.

Why this is a great menopause diet meal:

- Chicken is a lean protein source that can help maintain muscle mass and support overall health during menopause.
- Broccoli and bell peppers are rich in vitamins, minerals, and antioxidants that can help reduce inflammation and support menopausal women's well-being.
- The ginger and garlic in this dish provide additional anti-inflammatory benefits and may help alleviate some menopausal symptoms.
- Brown rice is a whole grain that provides complex carbohydrates, fiber, and B vitamins, which can help maintain energy levels and support overall health.
- This stir-fry is a well-balanced, nutrient-dense meal that is easy to prepare and can be enjoyed as part of a menopause-friendly diet

How would you rate this dish?

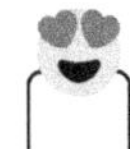 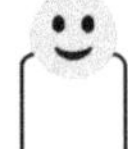  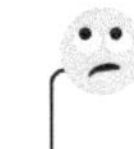 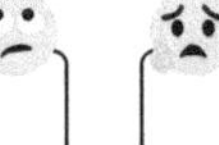

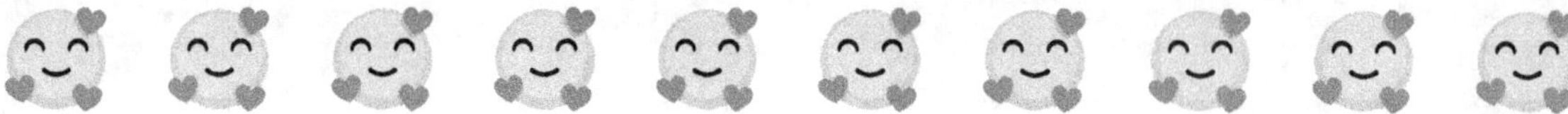

33. Baked Cod with Lemon and Herbs

Let's do that and fill in the time here

 Prep Time :　　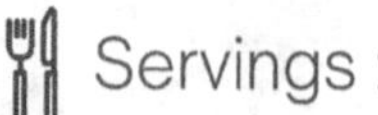 Cook Time :　　Servings :

Is this dish easy or difficult for you to make?

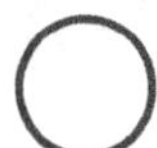 ◯　　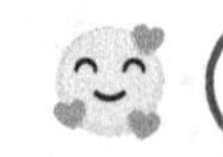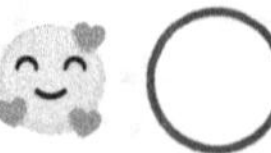 ◯

Write 5 friends with whom you want to share this dish

....

....

....

....

....

INGREDIENTS

- 1 lb cod fillets, about 4 pieces
- 2 tablespoons olive oil
- 2 tablespoons freshly squeezed lemon juice
- 2 garlic cloves, minced
- 2 tablespoons chopped fresh parsley
- 1 tablespoon chopped fresh dill (or 1 teaspoon dried dill)
- 1/2 teaspoon salt
- 1/4 teaspoon black pepper

1. Preheat your oven to 400°F (200°C).

2. In a small bowl, whisk together the olive oil, lemon juice, garlic, parsley, dill, salt, and pepper.

3. Place the cod fillets in a baking dish or on a parchment-lined baking sheet. Pour the lemon-herb mixture over the top of the fish, making sure to evenly coat the fillets.

4. Bake the cod for 12-15 minutes, or until the fish is opaque and flakes easily with a fork.

5. Serve the baked cod immediately, garnished with additional fresh parsley or dill if desired.

Why this is a great menopause diet meal:

- Cod is an excellent source of lean protein, which is important for maintaining muscle mass and overall health during menopause.
- Cod is also a good source of omega-3 fatty acids, which can help reduce inflammation and support heart health.
- The lemon and herbs in this recipe provide a flavorful way to prepare the cod without the need for heavy sauces or breading, keeping the dish light and healthy.
- Herbs like parsley and dill are rich in antioxidants, which can help protect against the oxidative stress associated with menopause.
- This baked cod dish is easy to prepare and can be served with a side of roasted vegetables or a fresh salad for a complete and balanced meal.

How would you rate this dish?

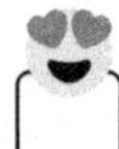 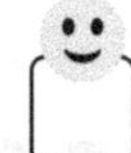 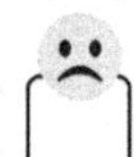 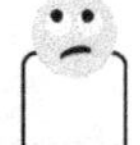 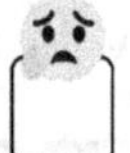

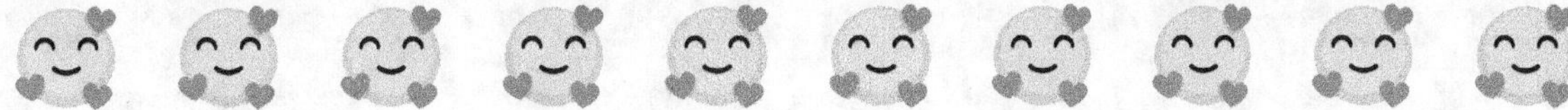

34. Stuffed Portobello Mushrooms with Quinoa and Spinach

Let's do that and fill in the time here

 Prep Time :

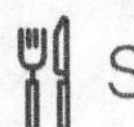 Cook Time :

Servings :

Is this dish easy or difficult for you to make?

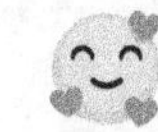 ◯   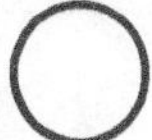 ◯

Write 5 friends with whom you want to share this dish

....

....

....

....

....

INGREDIENTS

- 4 large portobello mushroom caps, stems removed and chopped
- 1 cup cooked quinoa
- 1 cup fresh spinach, chopped
- 1/4 cup crumbled feta cheese
- 2 tablespoons olive oil
- 2 garlic cloves, minced
- 1/4 teaspoon dried oregano
- 1/4 teaspoon salt
- 1/8 teaspoon black pepper

1. Preheat your oven to 400°F (200°C).

2. In a medium bowl, combine the chopped mushroom stems, cooked quinoa, spinach, feta cheese, 1 tablespoon of the olive oil, garlic, oregano, salt, and pepper. Mix well.

3. Brush the portobello mushroom caps with the remaining 1 tablespoon of olive oil and place them on a baking sheet or in a baking dish.

4. Spoon the quinoa-spinach mixture evenly into the mushroom caps, packing it down gently.

5. Bake the stuffed mushrooms for 15-20 minutes, or until the mushrooms are tender and the filling is heated through.

6. Serve the Stuffed Portobello Mushrooms with Quinoa and Spinach warm.

Why this is a great menopause diet meal:

- Portobello mushrooms are a good source of vitamin D, which is important for bone health during menopause.
- Quinoa is a nutrient-dense whole grain that provides complex carbohydrates, protein, and fiber to help keep you feeling full and satisfied.
- Spinach is rich in vitamins, minerals, and antioxidants that can help support overall health during menopause.
- Feta cheese is a good source of calcium, which is crucial for maintaining

How would you rate this dish?

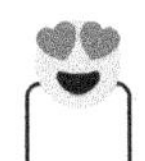 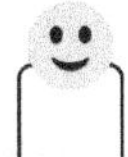 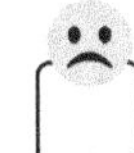 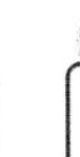 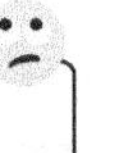 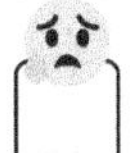

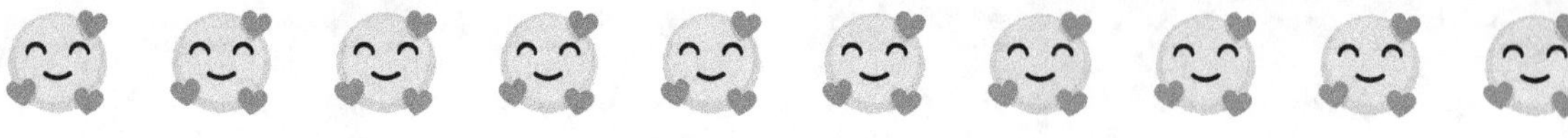

35. Turkey Chili with Black Beans

 Prep Time : 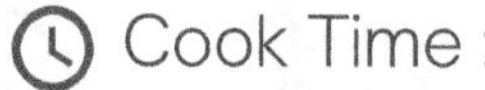 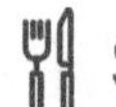 Cook Time : Servings :

Is this dish easy or difficult for you to make?

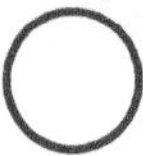 ◯ 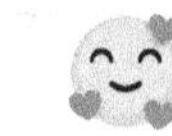 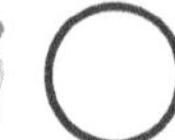 ◯

Write 5 friends with whom you want to share this dish

INGREDIENTS

- 1 lb ground turkey
- 1 tablespoon olive oil
- 1 onion, diced
- 3 garlic cloves, minced
- 2 tablespoons chili powder
- 1 teaspoon ground cumin
- 1 teaspoon dried oregano
- 1/2 teaspoon smoked paprika
- 1/4 teaspoon cayenne pepper (optional)
- 1 (15 oz) can black beans, drained and rinsed
- 1 (15 oz) can diced tomatoes
- 1 (6 oz) can tomato paste
- 1 cup low-sodium chicken or vegetable broth
- Salt and black pepper to taste
- Chopped fresh cilantro for garnish (optional)

1. In a large pot or Dutch oven, heat the olive oil over medium-high heat. Add the ground turkey and cook, breaking it up with a wooden spoon, until browned and cooked through, about 5-7 minutes.

2. Add the diced onion and sauté for 3-4 minutes, until translucent. Add the minced garlic and cook for an additional minute, stirring constantly.

3. Stir in the chili powder, cumin, oregano, smoked paprika, and cayenne pepper (if using). Cook for 1-2 minutes to toast the spices.

4. Add the black beans, diced tomatoes, tomato paste, and chicken or vegetable broth. Stir to combine.

5. Bring the chili to a simmer and let it cook for 20-25 minutes, stirring occasionally, until the flavors have melded and the chili has thickened.

6. Season the chili with salt and black pepper to taste.

7. Serve the Turkey Chili with Black Beans hot, garnished with chopped fresh cilantro if desired. Enjoy with a side of whole grain crackers or a fresh salad.

Enjoy this delicious and nutritious Turkey Chili with Black Beans as a comforting and satisfying addition to your menopause diet.

How would you rate this dish?

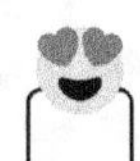 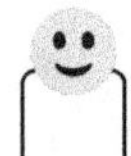 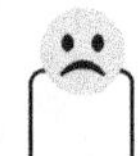 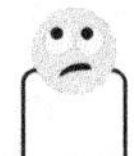 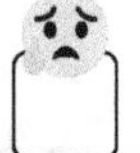

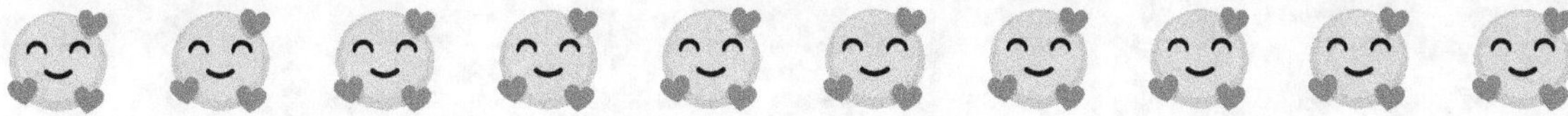

36. Spaghetti Squash with Marinara Sauce and Ground Turkey

 Prep Time :

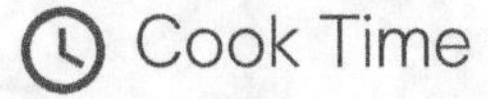 Cook Time :

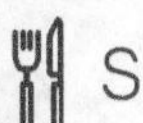 Servings :

Write 5 friends with whom you want to share this dish

....
....
....
....
....

Is this dish easy or difficult for you to make?

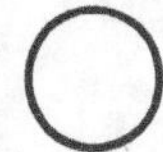 ◯   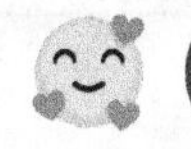 ◯

INGREDIENTS

- 1 medium spaghetti squash, halved lengthwise and seeds removed
- 1 lb ground turkey
- 1 tablespoon olive oil
- 1 onion, diced
- 3 garlic cloves, minced
- 1 (28 oz) can crushed tomatoes
- 2 tablespoons tomato paste
- 1 teaspoon dried oregano
- 1/2 teaspoon dried basil
- 1/4 teaspoon red pepper flakes (optional)
- Salt and pepper to taste
- Grated Parmesan cheese (optional)

1. Preheat the oven to 400°F (200°C). Place the spaghetti squash halves cut-side down on a baking sheet. Bake for 40-50 minutes, or until the squash is tender and easily shreds with a fork.

2. In a large skillet, cook the ground turkey over medium-high heat, breaking it up with a wooden spoon, until browned and cooked through, about 5-7 minutes. Transfer the cooked turkey to a plate and set aside.

3. In the same skillet, heat the olive oil over medium heat. Add the diced onion and sauté for 3-4 minutes until translucent. Add the minced garlic and cook for an additional minute, stirring constantly.

4. Stir in the crushed tomatoes, tomato paste, oregano, basil, and red pepper flakes (if using). Season with salt and pepper to taste. Bring the sauce to a simmer and let it cook for 10-15 minutes, stirring occasionally, to allow the flavors to meld.

5. Add the cooked ground turkey back to the sauce and stir to combine.

6. Use a fork to shred the cooked spaghetti squash into strands. Divide the squash strands among plates or bowls and top with the marinara sauce and turkey mixture.

7. Optionally, sprinkle grated Parmesan cheese over the top.

Enjoy this Spaghetti Squash with Marinara Sauce and Ground Turkey as a delicious and nutritious meal for your menopause diet.

How would you rate this dish?

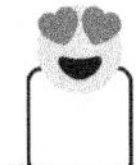 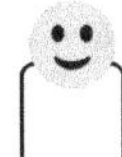 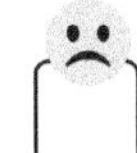 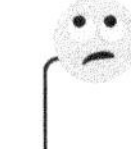 

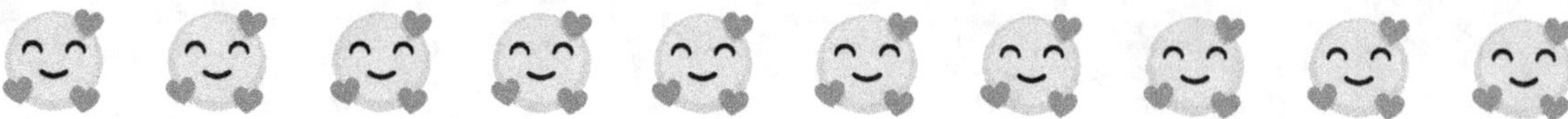

37. Shrimp Skewers with Vegetables

 Prep Time :   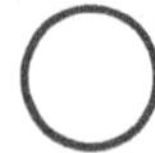 Cook Time :   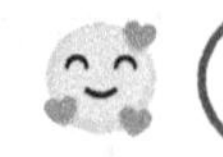 Servings :

Is this dish easy or difficult for you to make?

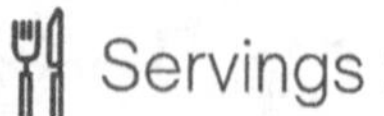 ◯   ◯

Write 5 friends with whom you want to share this dish

....

....

....

....

....

INGREDIENTS

- 1 lb large shrimp, peeled and deveined
- 1 red bell pepper, cut into 1-inch pieces
- 1 zucchini, cut into 1-inch pieces
- 1 red onion, cut into 1-inch pieces
- 2 tablespoons olive oil
- 2 tablespoons lemon juice
- 2 garlic cloves, minced
- 1 teaspoon dried oregano
- 1/2 teaspoon salt
- 1/4 teaspoon black pepper
- Wooden or metal skewers

1. If using wooden skewers, soak them in water for 30 minutes to prevent them from burning.

2. In a large bowl, combine the shrimp, bell pepper, zucchini, and red onion.

3. In a small bowl, whisk together the olive oil, lemon juice, garlic, oregano, salt, and black pepper.

4. Pour the marinade over the shrimp and vegetables and toss to coat everything evenly. Cover and refrigerate for 30 minutes to 1 hour.

5. Preheat your grill or grill pan to medium-high heat.

6. Thread the marinated shrimp and vegetables onto the skewers, alternating the ingredients.

7. Grill the skewers for 2-3 minutes per side, or until the shrimp are opaque and the vegetables are tender-crisp.

8. Serve the Shrimp Skewers with Vegetables immediately.

Why this is a great menopause diet meal:

- Shrimp is a lean protein source that can help maintain muscle mass and support overall health during menopause.

- The vegetables, such as bell peppers, zucchini, and onions, are rich in vitamins, minerals, and antioxidants that can help reduce inflammation and support menopausal women's well-being.

How would you rate this dish?

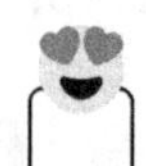 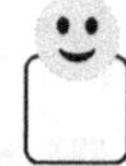 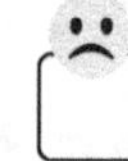 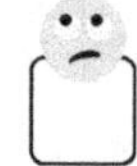 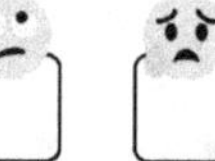

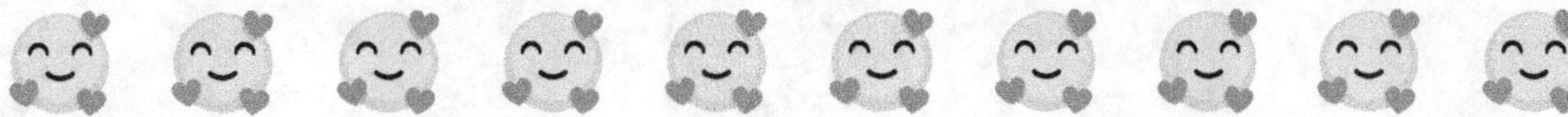

38. Vegetable Stir-Fry with Tofu

Let's do that and fill in the time here

🕐 Prep Time :　　🕐 Cook Time :　　🍴 Servings :

Write 5 friends with whom you want to share this dish

....
....
....
....
....

Is this dish easy or difficult for you to make?

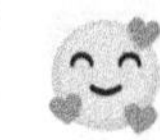 ◯　　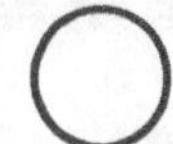 ◯

INGREDIENTS

- 1 block (14 oz) extra-firm tofu, drained and cubed
- 2 tablespoons low-sodium soy sauce or tamari
- 1 tablespoon sesame oil
- 2 tablespoons olive oil
- 3 cups mixed vegetables (such as broccoli, bell peppers, snow peas, and mushrooms), chopped
- 3 garlic cloves, minced
- 1 tablespoon grated fresh ginger
- 2 tablespoons rice vinegar
- 1 tablespoon honey or maple syrup
- 1/4 teaspoon red pepper flakes (optional)
- Salt and pepper to taste
- Cooked brown rice, for serving

How would you rate this dish?

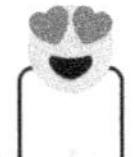   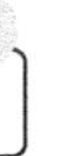 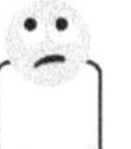 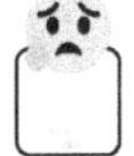

1. In a medium bowl, toss the cubed tofu with the soy sauce and sesame oil. Set aside.

2. Heat the olive oil in a large skillet or wok over high heat. Add the mixed vegetables and stir-fry for 3-4 minutes, until they start to soften.

3. Add the garlic and ginger to the skillet and cook for 1 minute, stirring constantly, until fragrant.

4. Add the marinated tofu to the skillet and continue to stir-fry for 5-7 minutes, until the tofu is lightly browned and the vegetables are tender-crisp.

5. Stir in the rice vinegar, honey or maple syrup, and red pepper flakes (if using). Season with salt and pepper to taste.

6. Serve the Vegetable Stir-Fry with Tofu immediately over cooked brown rice.

Why this is a great menopause diet meal:

- Tofu is a plant-based protein source that can help maintain muscle mass and support overall health during menopause.

- The variety of vegetables in this dish provide a wide range of vitamins, minerals, and antioxidants that can help reduce inflammation and support menopausal women's well-being.

- Ginger and garlic have anti-inflammatory properties that may help alleviate some menopausal symptoms.

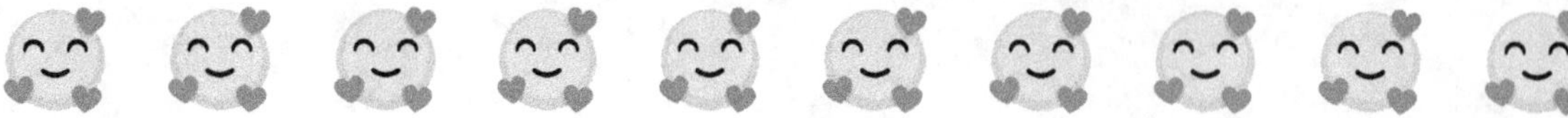

39. Grilled Lamb Chops with Mint Yogurt Sauce

Let's do that and fill in the time here

 Prep Time : 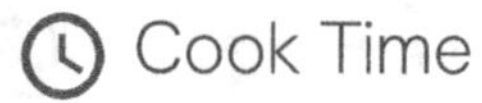

 Cook Time :

Servings :

Is this dish easy or difficult for you to make?

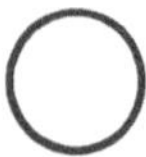 ○   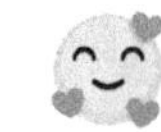  ○

Write 5 friends with whom you want to share this dish

....

....

....

....

....

INGREDIENTS

- 8 lamb chops (about 1-1.5 lbs)
- 2 tablespoons olive oil
- 1 teaspoon dried oregano
- 1/2 teaspoon salt
- 1/4 teaspoon black pepper

For the Mint Yogurt Sauce:
- 1 cup plain Greek yogurt
- 2 tablespoons chopped fresh mint
- 1 tablespoon lemon juice
- 1 garlic clove, minced
- 1/4 teaspoon salt

1. Preheat your grill or grill pan to medium-high heat.

2. In a small bowl, combine the olive oil, oregano, salt, and black pepper. Rub this mixture all over the lamb chops.

3. Grill the lamb chops for 3-4 minutes per side, or until they reach the desired level of doneness. Transfer the grilled chops to a plate and let them rest for 5 minutes.

4. In a separate bowl, mix together the Greek yogurt, chopped mint, lemon juice, garlic, and salt for the mint yogurt sauce.

5. Serve the grilled lamb chops warm, drizzled with the mint yogurt sauce.

Why this is a great menopause diet meal:

- Lamb is a lean protein source that can help maintain muscle mass and support overall health during menopause.
- The mint yogurt sauce provides a refreshing and flavorful accompaniment to the lamb, without the need for heavy or creamy sauces.
- Yogurt is a good source of calcium, which is important for maintaining bone health during menopause.
- Mint and lemon juice in the sauce can help aid digestion and provide anti-inflammatory benefits.
- This grilled lamb dish is easy to prepare and can be served with a side of roasted vegetables or a fresh salad for a complete and balanced menopause-friendly meal.

How would you rate this dish?

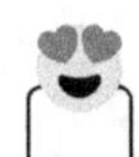 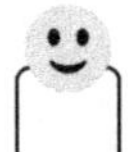  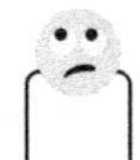 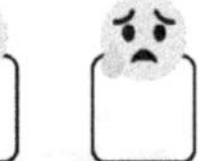

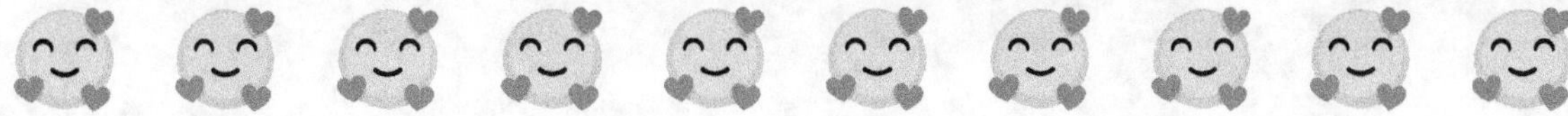

40. Baked Chicken Thighs with Sweet Potatoes and Brussel Sprouts

Let's do that and fill in the time here

Prep Time :

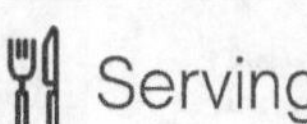

Cook Time :

Servings :

Write 5 friends with whom you want to share this dish

....

....

....

....

....

Is this dish easy or difficult for you to make?

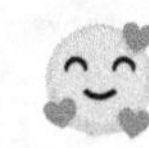 ◯

 ◯

INGREDIENTS

- 8 bone-in, skin-on chicken thighs
- 2 medium sweet potatoes, peeled and cubed
- 1 lb Brussels sprouts, trimmed and halved
- 2 tablespoons olive oil
- 1 teaspoon dried thyme
- 1 teaspoon paprika
- 1/2 teaspoon garlic powder
- 1/2 teaspoon salt
- 1/4 teaspoon black pepper

1. Preheat your oven to 400°F (200°C).

2. In a large bowl, combine the chicken thighs, cubed sweet potatoes, and Brussels sprouts. Drizzle with the olive oil and sprinkle with the thyme, paprika, garlic powder, salt, and black pepper. Toss to coat everything evenly.

3. Arrange the chicken, sweet potatoes, and Brussels sprouts in a single layer on a large baking sheet or in a large baking dish.

4. Bake for 35-40 minutes, or until the chicken is cooked through (internal temperature reaches 165°F/74°C) and the vegetables are tender.

5. Serve the Baked Chicken Thighs with Sweet Potatoes and Brussels Sprouts immediately.

Why this is a great menopause diet meal:

- Chicken thighs are a good source of lean protein, which can help maintain muscle mass and support overall health during menopause.
- Sweet potatoes are rich in beta-carotene, vitamin C, and fiber, all of which can help support menopausal women's well-being.
- Brussels sprouts are a cruciferous vegetable that contains antioxidants and may help reduce inflammation associated with menopause.
- The combination of protein, complex carbohydrates, and fiber in this dish can help keep you feeling full and satisfied.
- This one-pan baked meal is easy to prepare and can be served with a side of whole grain bread or a fresh salad for a complete and balanced menopause-friendly meal

How would you rate this dish?

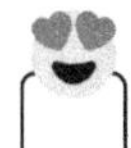 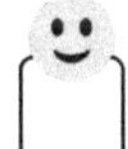 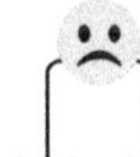 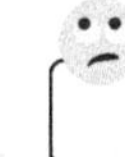 

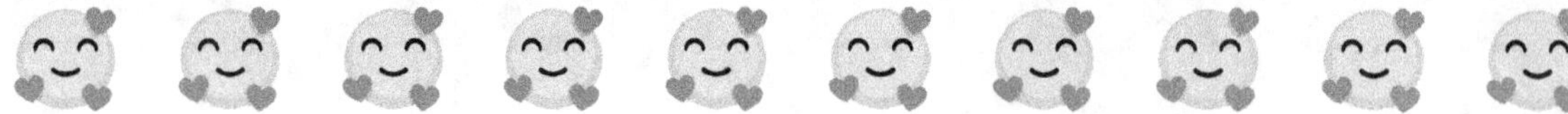

41. Dark Chocolate with Almonds

 Prep Time :   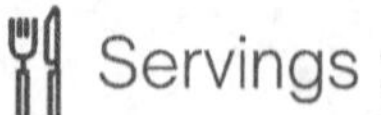 Cook Time :   Servings :

Is this dish easy or difficult for you to make?

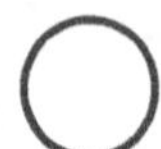  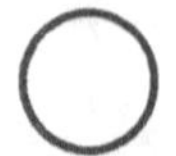

Write 5 friends with whom you want to share this dish

....

....

....

....

....

INGREDIENTS

- 4 oz dark chocolate (70% cacao or higher), chopped
- 1/2 cup raw, unsalted almonds

1. In a microwave-safe bowl, melt the chopped dark chocolate in the microwave, stirring every 30 seconds, until smooth and fully melted.

2. Add the raw almonds to the melted chocolate and stir to coat the almonds evenly.

3. Spread the chocolate-coated almonds in a single layer on a parchment-lined baking sheet or plate.

4. Refrigerate the chocolate-covered almonds for 15-20 minutes, or until the chocolate has hardened.

5. Once set, break the chocolate-covered almonds into individual pieces or small clusters.

6. Store the Dark Chocolate with Almonds in an airtight container in the refrigerator for up to 2 weeks.

Why this is a great menopause diet snack:

- Dark chocolate is rich in antioxidants and may help improve mood and cognitive function, which can be beneficial for menopausal women.
- Almonds are a good source of healthy fats, protein, fiber, and magnesium, all of which are important for menopausal women's health.
- The combination of dark chocolate and almonds provides a satisfying, nutrient-dense snack that can help curb cravings and provide a boost of energy.
- This simple recipe allows you to control the portion size and quality of the ingredients, making it a healthier alternative to store-bought chocolate-covered nuts

How would you rate this dish?

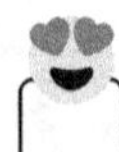 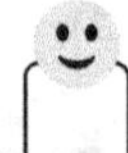 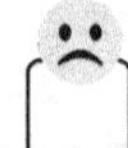 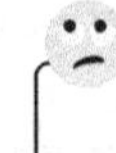 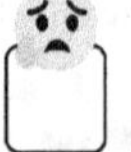

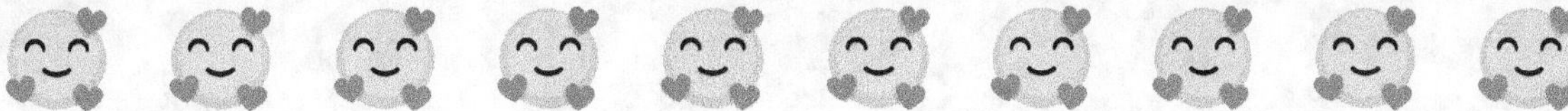

42. Chia Seed Pudding with Coconut Milk and Mango

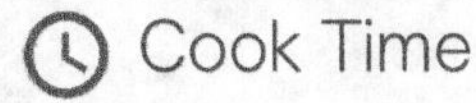 Prep Time :   Cook Time :   Servings :

Is this dish easy or difficult for you to make?

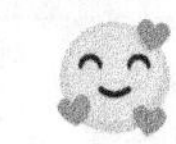 ◯   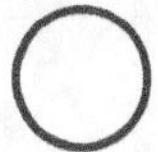 ◯

INGREDIENTS

- 1 cup unsweetened coconut milk
- 1/4 cup chia seeds
- 2 tablespoons honey or maple syrup (optional)
- 1 teaspoon vanilla extract
- 1 cup diced fresh mango
- Toasted coconut flakes for garnish (optional)

1. In a medium bowl, whisk together the coconut milk, chia seeds, honey/maple syrup (if using), and vanilla extract until well combined.

2. Cover the bowl and refrigerate for at least 4 hours, or overnight, stirring occasionally, until the chia seeds have thickened the mixture into a pudding-like consistency.

3. When ready to serve, divide the chia seed pudding evenly among 4 serving bowls or glasses.

4. Top each serving with 1/4 cup of diced fresh mango.

5. Optionally, sprinkle toasted coconut flakes over the top of the pudding. Serve chilled.

Why this is a great menopause diet dessert:

- Chia seeds are an excellent source of omega-3 fatty acids, fiber, and protein, all of which are important for menopausal women's health.
- Coconut milk is a dairy-free, nutrient-rich alternative to regular milk, providing healthy fats and a creamy texture.
- Mangoes are a good source of vitamins C and A, as well as antioxidants that can help reduce inflammation and support overall well-being during menopause.
- The natural sweetness from the honey or maple syrup (if used) provides a touch of sweetness without the need for added sugars.
- This dessert is easy to prepare, refreshing, and can be enjoyed as a healthy snack or light dessert.

How would you rate this dish?

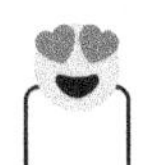 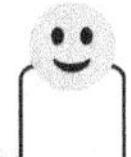  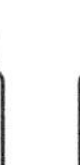 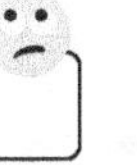

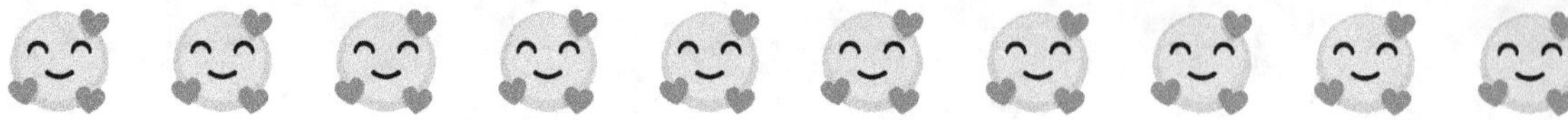

43. Frozen Yogurt with Fresh Berries

 Prep Time :   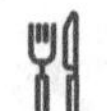 Cook Time :   Servings :

Is this dish easy or difficult for you to make?

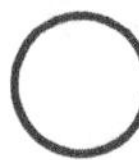 ◯   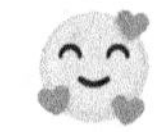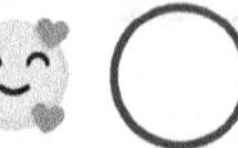 ◯

Write 5 friends with whom you want to share this dish

INGREDIENTS

- 2 cups plain Greek yogurt
- 1/4 cup honey or maple syrup
- 1 teaspoon vanilla extract
- 1 cup mixed fresh berries (such as raspberries, blueberries, and strawberries)

1. In a medium bowl, whisk together the Greek yogurt, honey or maple syrup, and vanilla extract until well combined.

2. Pour the yogurt mixture into a shallow baking dish or a freezer-safe container.

3. Place the dish or container in the freezer and freeze for 2-3 hours, stirring the mixture with a fork every 30 minutes, until it reaches a soft, scoopable consistency.

4. Scoop the frozen yogurt into serving bowls or cups.

5. Top each serving with a generous amount of the fresh mixed berries. Serve the Frozen Yogurt with Fresh Berries immediately.

Why this is a great menopause diet dessert:

- Greek yogurt is a good source of protein, which can help maintain muscle mass and support overall health during menopause.
- The probiotics in yogurt can also help support gut health, which is important for menopausal women.
- Berries are rich in antioxidants, vitamins, and fiber, which can help reduce inflammation and support menopausal women's well-being.
- The natural sweetness from the honey or maple syrup provides a touch of sweetness without the need for added sugars.
- This frozen yogurt dessert is light, refreshing, and can be enjoyed as a healthy treat or snack during menopause.

How would you rate this dish?

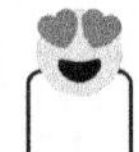  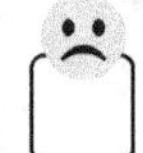 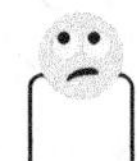 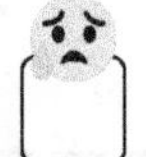

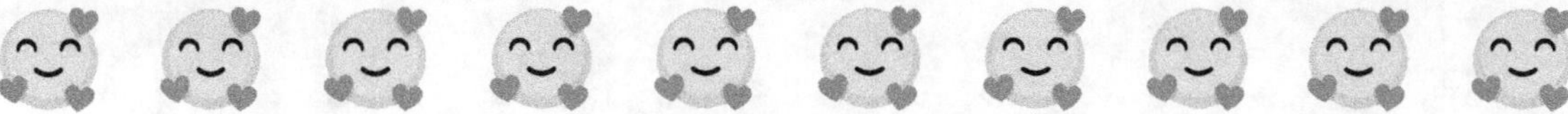

44. Baked Apples with Cinnamon and Walnuts

 Prep Time : 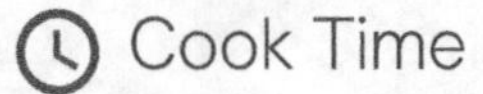 Cook Time :  Servings :

Write 5 friends with whom you want to share this dish

Is this dish easy or difficult for you to make?

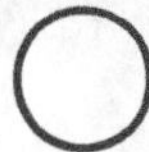 ◯   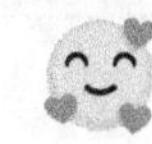 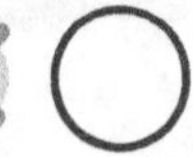 ◯

INGREDIENTS

- 4 medium-sized apples (such as Honeycrisp or Gala)
- 1/4 cup chopped walnuts
- 2 tablespoons brown sugar
- 1 teaspoon ground cinnamon
- 1/4 teaspoon ground nutmeg
- 2 tablespoons unsalted butter, softened
- 1/4 cup water or apple cider

1. Preheat your oven to 375°F (190°C).

2. Core the apples, leaving about 1/2 inch of the bottom intact. Use a paring knife or melon baller to carefully scoop out the core, creating a well in the center of each apple.

3. In a small bowl, mix together the chopped walnuts, brown sugar, cinnamon, and nutmeg.

4. Stuff the walnut-spice mixture into the center of each cored apple. Top each apple with a small pat of the softened butter.

5. Place the stuffed apples in a baking dish and pour the water or apple cider into the bottom of the dish.

6. Bake the apples for 30-40 minutes, or until they are tender when pierced with a fork and the filling is bubbly.

7. Serve the Baked Apples with Cinnamon and Walnuts warm, with the cooking liquid spooned over the top.

Why this is a great menopause diet dessert:

- Apples are a good source of fiber, which can help regulate digestion and support gut health during menopause.

- Walnuts are rich in omega-3 fatty acids, which can help reduce inflammation and support overall health.

- Cinnamon and nutmeg have anti-inflammatory properties that may help alleviate some menopausal symptoms.

How would you rate this dish?

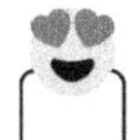 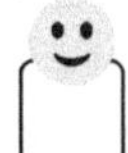 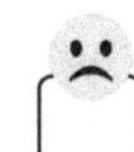 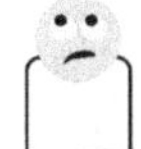 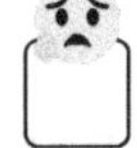

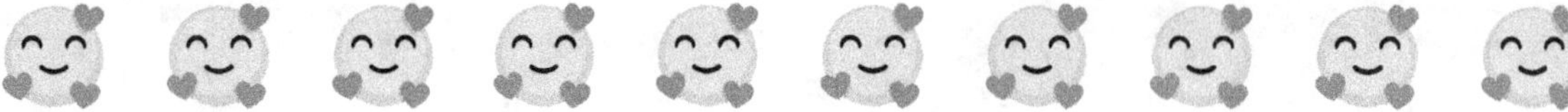

45. Banana Ice Cream with Peanut Butter

 Prep Time : 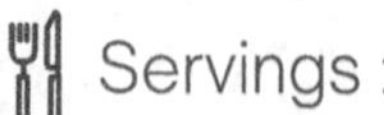 Cook Time : Servings :

Write 5 friends with whom you want to share this dish

....
....
....
....
....

INGREDIENTS

- 3 ripe bananas, peeled and frozen
- 2 tablespoons creamy peanut butter
- 1 tablespoon honey or maple syrup (optional)
- 1/4 teaspoon vanilla extract

Is this dish easy or difficult for you to make?

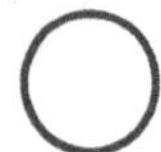 ◯ 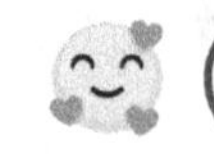 ◯

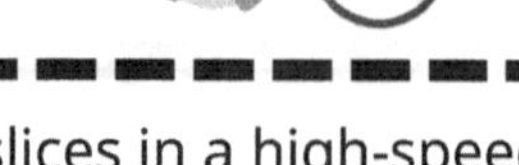

1. Place the frozen banana slices in a high-speed blender or food processor.

2. Add the peanut butter, honey or maple syrup (if using), and vanilla extract.

3. Blend or process the ingredients until smooth and creamy, stopping to scrape down the sides as needed. The mixture should have a soft, ice cream-like consistency.

4. Serve the Banana Ice Cream with Peanut Butter immediately, or transfer it to an airtight container and freeze for 30-60 minutes for a firmer texture.

Why this is a great menopause diet dessert:

- Bananas are a good source of potassium, which can help regulate blood pressure and support overall health during menopause.
- Peanut butter provides healthy fats and protein, which can help keep you feeling full and satisfied.
- The natural sweetness from the bananas and optional honey or maple syrup provides a touch of sweetness without the need for added sugars.
- This dessert is dairy-free, making it a great option for those who are lactose intolerant or prefer a plant-based treat.
- The combination of the creamy banana "ice cream" and the peanut butter creates a delicious and satisfying dessert that can be enjoyed as part of a balanced menopause diet.

Enjoy this Banana Ice Cream with Peanut Butter as a healthy and indulgent treat during menopause.

How would you rate this dish?

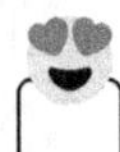 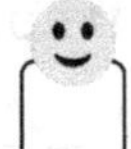 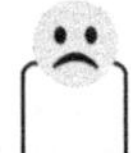 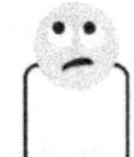 

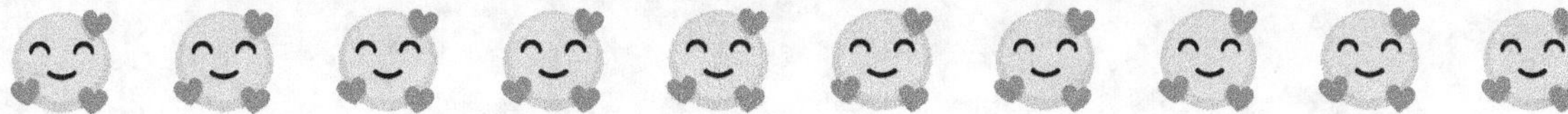

46. Oatmeal Cookies with Dark Chocolate Chips

 Prep Time :    Cook Time :   Servings :

Write 5 friends with whom you want to share this dish

Is this dish easy or difficult for you to make?

 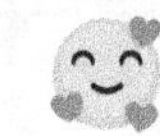 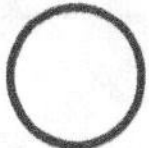 ◯   ◯

INGREDIENTS

- 1 cup (2 sticks) unsalted butter, softened
- 1 cup brown sugar
- 1 egg
- 1 teaspoon vanilla extract
- 1 1/2 cups old-fashioned oats
- 1 1/4 cups whole wheat flour
- 1 teaspoon baking soda
- 1/2 teaspoon ground cinnamon
- 1/4 teaspoon salt
- 1 cup dark chocolate chips

1. Preheat your oven to 350°F (175°C). Line a baking sheet with parchment paper.

2. In a large bowl, cream the softened butter and brown sugar together until light and fluffy, about 2-3 minutes.

3. Beat in the egg and vanilla extract until well combined.

4. In a separate bowl, whisk together the old-fashioned oats, whole wheat flour, baking soda, cinnamon, and salt.

5. Gradually add the dry ingredients to the wet ingredients, mixing until just combined. Fold in the dark chocolate chips.

6. Scoop rounded tablespoons of the dough onto the prepared baking sheet, spacing them about 2 inches apart.

7. Bake for 10-12 minutes, or until the cookies are lightly golden around the edges. Be careful not to overbake.

8. Allow the cookies to cool on the baking sheet for 5 minutes before transferring them to a wire rack to cool completely.

Enjoy these Oatmeal Cookies with Dark Chocolate Chips as a delicious and nutritious snack or dessert option during menopause.

How would you rate this dish?

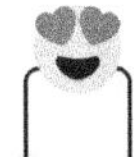 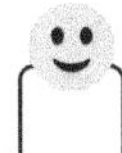 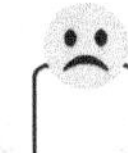 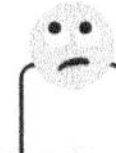 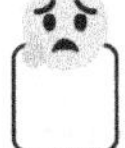

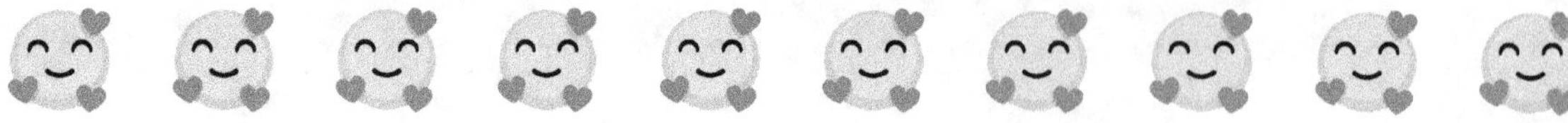

47. Fruit Salad with Honey and Mint

 Prep Time :  Cook Time : Servings :

Write 5 friends with whom you want to share this dish

....

....

....

....

....

Is this dish easy or difficult for you to make?

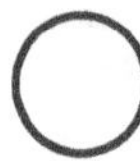 ○   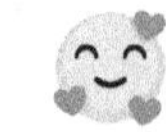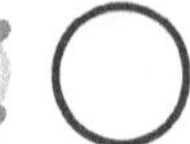 ○

INGREDIENTS

- 2 cups mixed fresh fruit (such as diced apples, grapes, pineapple, strawberries, blueberries, etc.)
- 2 tablespoons honey
- 1-2 tablespoons chopped fresh mint leaves

1. In a medium bowl, combine the mixed fresh fruit.

2. Drizzle the honey over the fruit and gently toss to coat.

3. Sprinkle the chopped fresh mint leaves over the top.

4. Gently stir to combine.

5. Chill the fruit salad in the refrigerator for at least 30 minutes before serving to allow the flavors to meld.

6. Serve chilled. The honey and mint provide a lovely sweet and refreshing contrast to the juicy fruit.

Enjoy this simple, healthy, and flavorful fruit salad! The honey and mint make it a perfect light dessert or side dish.

How would you rate this dish?

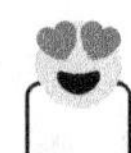 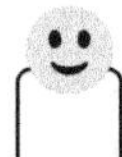 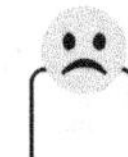 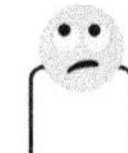 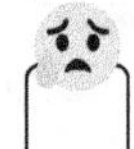

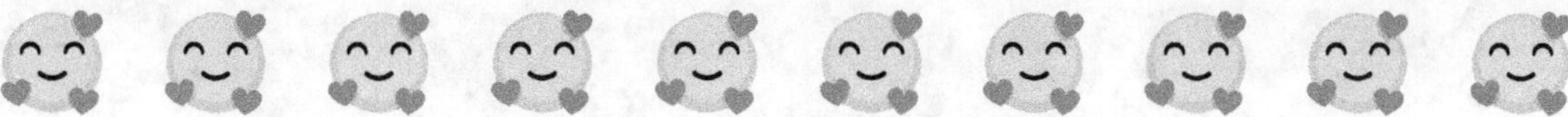

48. Greek Yogurt with Honey and Nuts

Let's do that and fill in the time here

 Prep Time :   Cook Time :   Servings :

Write 5 friends with whom you want to share this dish

....
....
....
....
....

Is this dish easy or difficult for you to make?

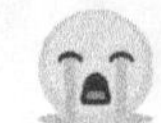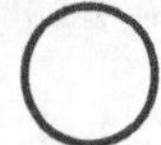 ◯   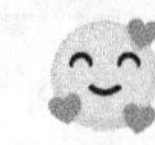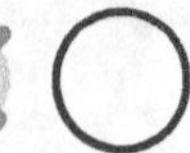 ◯

INGREDIENTS

- 1 cup plain Greek yogurt
- 1-2 tablespoons honey
- 2-3 tablespoons chopped nuts (such as walnuts, almonds, or pistachios)
- Optional: Fresh berries or sliced fruit

1. In a bowl or parfait glass, layer the Greek yogurt and honey. Stir gently to swirl the honey into the yogurt.

2. Top the yogurt with the chopped nuts.

3. If desired, add a layer of fresh berries or sliced fruit on top of the nuts.. Serve chilled.

Why this is a great menopause diet option:

- Greek yogurt is high in protein, which can help maintain muscle mass and bone health during menopause.

- Honey provides natural sweetness and contains antioxidants.

- Nuts are a good source of healthy fats, fiber, and minerals like magnesium, which can help manage menopausal symptoms.

- The combination of protein, healthy fats, and fiber helps promote feelings of fullness and stable blood sugar levels.

This simple parfait makes for a nutritious and satisfying breakfast, snack, or light dessert that can be easily customized with different fruit and nut combinations. It's a great way to incorporate nutrient-dense foods into a menopause-friendly diet.

How would you rate this dish?

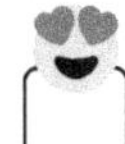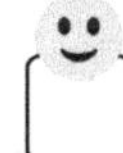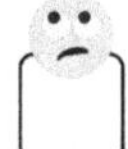

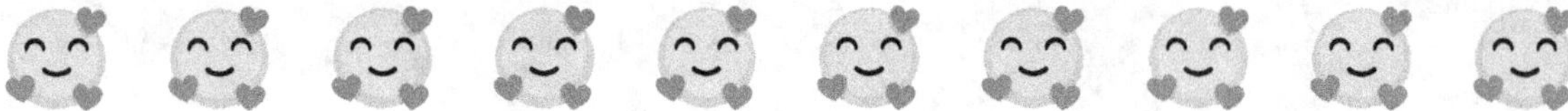

49. Chia Pudding with Almond Milk and Berries

Let's do that and fill in the time here

 Prep Time : 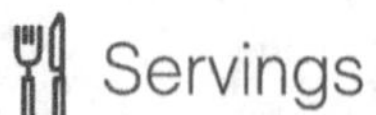 Cook Time : Servings :

Write 5 friends with whom you want to share this dish

....

....

....

....

....

Is this dish easy or difficult for you to make?

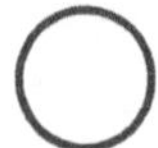 ◯ 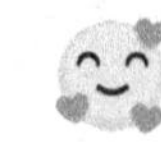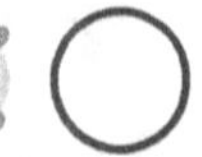 ◯

INGREDIENTS

- 1 cup unsweetened almond milk
- 1/4 cup chia seeds
- 1 tablespoon honey or maple syrup (optional)
- 1 teaspoon vanilla extract
- 1 cup mixed fresh or frozen berries (such as raspberries, blueberries, and strawberries)

1. In a medium bowl, whisk together the almond milk, chia seeds, honey or maple syrup (if using), and vanilla extract until well combined.

2. Cover the bowl and refrigerate for at least 4 hours, or overnight, stirring occasionally, until the chia seeds have thickened the mixture into a pudding-like consistency.

3. When ready to serve, divide the chia pudding evenly among 4 serving bowls or glasses.

4. Top each serving with 1/4 cup of the mixed berries.

5. Serve chilled.

Why this is a great menopause diet dessert:

- Chia seeds are an excellent source of omega-3 fatty acids, fiber, and protein, all of which are important for menopausal women's health.
- Almond milk is a dairy-free, low-calorie alternative that provides calcium and other essential nutrients.
- Berries are rich in antioxidants, vitamins, and fiber, which can help reduce inflammation and support overall well-being during menopause.
- The natural sweetness from the optional honey or maple syrup provides a touch of sweetness without the need for added sugars.
- This dessert is easy to prepare, refreshing, and can be enjoyed as a healthy snack or light dessert.

The Chia Pudding with Almond Milk and Berries is a delicious and nutritious option that can be a great addition to a menopause diet. Enjoy this flavorful and satisfying treat.

How would you rate this dish?

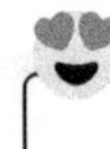 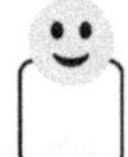 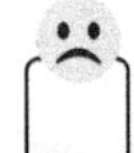 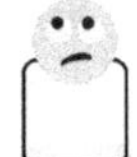 

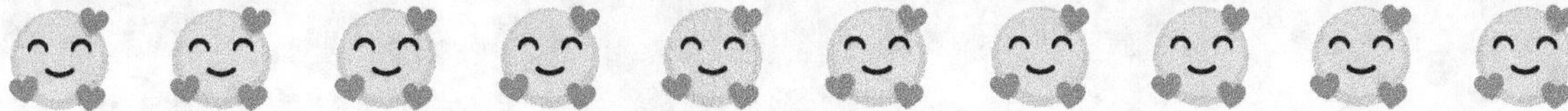

50. Homemade Granola Bars with Nuts and Seeds

 _Let's do that and fill in the time here_   Prep Time :   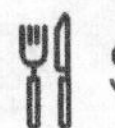 Cook Time :   Servings :

Is this dish easy or difficult for you to make?

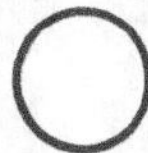 ◯   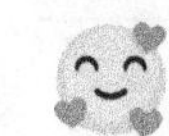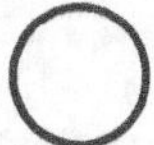 ◯

Write 5 friends with whom you want to share this dish

INGREDIENTS

- 2 cups old-fashioned rolled oats
- 1/2 cup chopped nuts (such as almonds, walnuts, pecans)
- 1/4 cup shelled sunflower seeds
- 1/4 cup shelled pumpkin seeds
- 1/4 cup unsweetened shredded coconut (optional)
- 1/4 cup honey
- 1/4 cup nut butter (such as peanut, almond or cashew butter)
- 1 teaspoon vanilla extract
- 1/4 teaspoon salt

1. Preheat the oven to 325°F. Line an 8x8 inch baking pan with parchment paper, leaving some overhang on the sides for easy removal.

2. In a large bowl, combine the rolled oats, chopped nuts, sunflower seeds, pumpkin seeds, and shredded coconut (if using). Stir to mix well.

3. In a small saucepan, heat the honey and nut butter over low heat, stirring constantly, until smooth and combined. Remove from heat and stir in the vanilla extract and salt.

4. Pour the honey-nut butter mixture over the dry ingredients and stir until everything is well coated.

5. Transfer the mixture to the prepared baking pan and press it down firmly and evenly with a spatula or your hands.

6. Bake for 20-25 minutes, until the edges are lightly golden brown.

7. Allow the granola bars to cool completely in the pan, then lift them out using the parchment paper overhang. Cut into bars or squares.

Store the homemade granola bars in an airtight container at room temperature for up to 1 week.

Enjoy these chewy, nutty, and wholesome granola bars as a healthy snack or on-the-go breakfast!

How would you rate this dish?

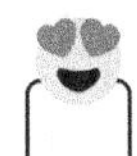 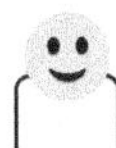 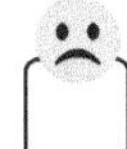 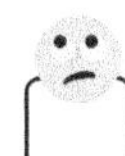 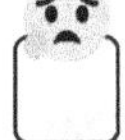

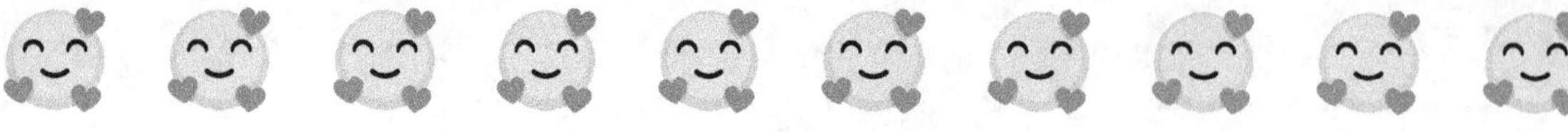

51. Berry and Spinach Smoothie

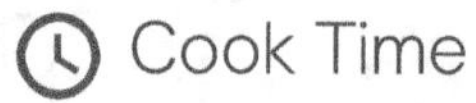 Prep Time :    Cook Time :   Servings :

Is this dish easy or difficult for you to make?

 ◯   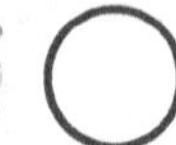 ◯

Write 5 friends with whom you want to share this dish

....

....

....

....

....

INGREDIENTS

- 1 cup fresh or frozen mixed berries (such as blueberries, raspberries, strawberries)
- 1 cup fresh spinach, packed
- 1 cup unsweetened almond milk (or other non-dairy milk)
- 1/2 cup plain Greek yogurt
- 1 tablespoon ground flaxseed
- 1 teaspoon honey (optional)

1. Add all the ingredients to a high-speed blender and blend until smooth and creamy.

2. Taste and adjust sweetener (honey) if needed.

3. Pour into a glass and enjoy immediately.

Why this is a great menopause diet option:

- Berries are rich in antioxidants, fiber, and phytonutrients that can help support overall health during menopause.

- Spinach is a nutrient-dense green packed with vitamins, minerals, and antioxidants that can help manage menopausal symptoms.

- Greek yogurt provides protein to help maintain muscle mass and bone health.

- Flaxseed is a good source of fiber, omega-3 fatty acids, and lignans, which may help alleviate some menopausal discomforts.

- The smoothie format makes it easy to consume a nutrient-dense meal or snack.

This Berry and Spinach Smoothie is a great way to incorporate more plant-based, fiber-rich, and anti-inflammatory foods into your menopause diet. It's refreshing, satisfying, and packed with beneficial nutrients to support your health during this transition.

How would you rate this dish?

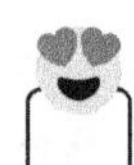 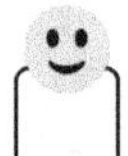 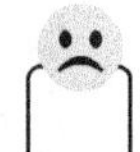 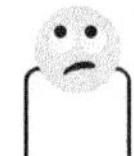 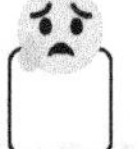

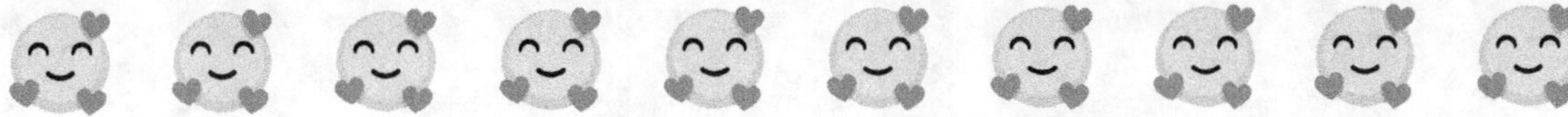

52. Green Detox Smoothie

 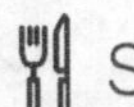

Prep Time :   Cook Time :   Servings :

Is this dish easy or difficult for you to make?

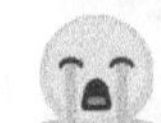 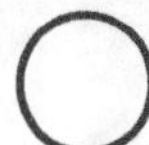 ◯   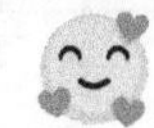  ◯

Write 5 friends with whom you want to share this dish

....
....
....
....

INGREDIENTS

- 1 cup spinach or kale, packed
- 1 cup unsweetened almond milk (or other non-dairy milk)
- 1/2 cup plain Greek yogurt
- 1 banana, frozen
- 1 tablespoon ground flaxseed
- 1 tablespoon honey (or maple syrup)
- 1/2 teaspoon ground ginger
- 1/4 teaspoon ground cinnamon

1. Add all the ingredients to a high-speed blender and blend until smooth and creamy.

2. Taste and adjust sweetener if needed.

3. Pour into a glass and enjoy immediately.

Why this is a great menopause diet option:

- Spinach and kale are nutrient-dense greens packed with vitamins, minerals, and antioxidants that can help support overall health during menopause.

- Greek yogurt provides protein to help maintain muscle mass.

- Flaxseed is a good source of fiber, omega-3 fatty acids, and lignans, which may help manage menopausal symptoms.

- Ginger and cinnamon are anti-inflammatory spices that can help alleviate some menopausal discomforts.

- Banana and honey/maple syrup add natural sweetness and carbohydrates for energy.

- The smoothie format makes it easy to consume a nutrient-dense meal or snack.

This Green Detox Smoothie is a great way to incorporate more plant-based, fiber-rich, and anti-inflammatory foods into your menopause diet. It's refreshing, satisfying, and packed with beneficial nutrients.

How would you rate this dish?

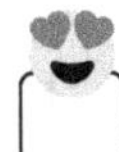 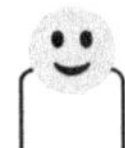 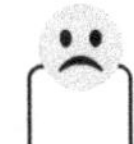 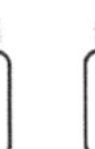 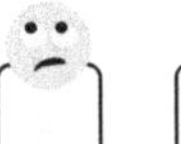 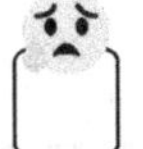

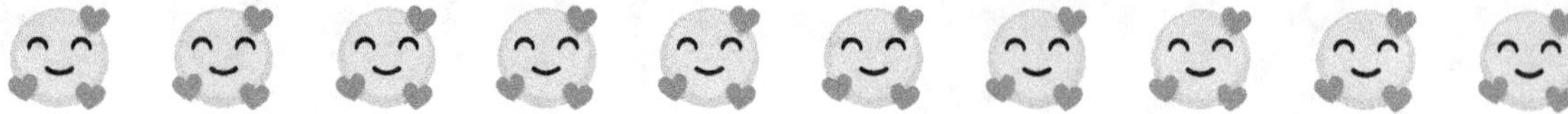

53. Peanut Butter and Banana Smoothie

 Prep Time :   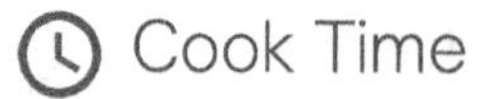 Cook Time :   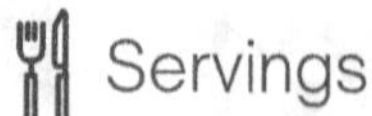 Servings :

Is this dish easy or difficult for you to make?

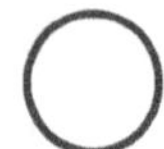 ◯   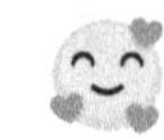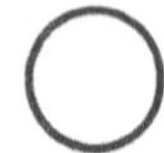 ◯

Write 5 friends with whom you want to share this dish

....

....

....

....

....

INGREDIENTS

- 1 ripe banana, frozen
- 2 tablespoons creamy peanut butter
- 1 cup unsweetened almond milk (or milk of your choice)
- 1/2 cup plain Greek yogurt
- 1 tablespoon honey (optional)
- 1/2 teaspoon vanilla extract
- Pinch of cinnamon (optional)

1. Add all the ingredients to a high-speed blender.

2. Blend on high speed until the mixture is smooth and creamy, about 1 minute.

3. Taste and adjust sweetener (honey) if desired.

4. Pour the smoothie into a glass and enjoy immediately.

Why this smoothie is a great choice:

- Banana provides natural sweetness, fiber, and potassium.

- Peanut butter adds healthy fats, protein, and a creamy texture.

- Greek yogurt boosts the protein content, making this smoothie more filling and satisfying.

- Almond milk is a great dairy-free option that's low in calories and high in nutrients.

- Honey (if used) provides a natural sweetener.

- Cinnamon adds a warm, comforting flavor and may have anti-inflammatory properties.

This Peanut Butter and Banana Smoothie is a delicious and nutritious way to start your day or enjoy as a healthy snack. The combination of protein, healthy fats, and carbohydrates makes it a well-balanced and satisfying option.

How would you rate this dish?

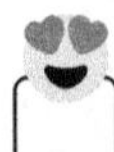   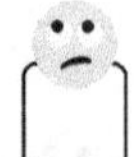 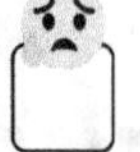

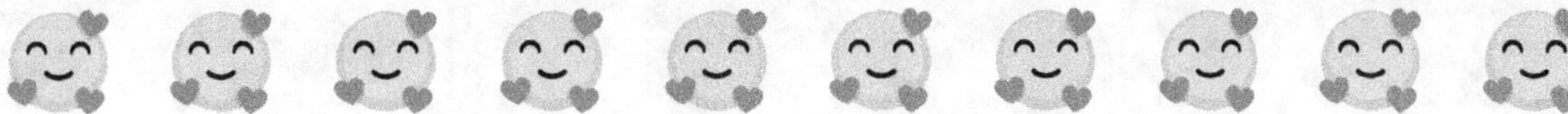

54. Mango and Turmeric Smoothie

Let's do that and fill in the time here

 Prep Time :  Cook Time : Servings :

Is this dish easy or difficult for you to make?

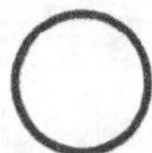 ◯  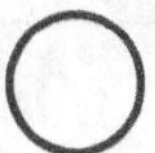 ◯

Write 5 friends with whom you want to share this dish

....

....

....

....

....

INGREDIENTS

- 1 cup frozen mango chunks
- 1 cup unsweetened almond milk
- 1 tablespoon ground turmeric
- 1 tablespoon honey or maple syrup (optional)
- 1 teaspoon ground ginger
- 1/2 teaspoon ground cinnamon
- 1/4 teaspoon black pepper

1. In a high-speed blender, combine the frozen mango chunks, almond milk, turmeric, honey or maple syrup (if using), ginger, cinnamon, and black pepper.

2. Blend on high speed until the mixture is smooth and creamy, about 1-2 minutes.

3. Pour the Mango and Turmeric Smoothie into a glass and enjoy immediately.

Why this is a great menopause diet smoothie:

- Mango is a good source of vitamins C and A, which can help support the immune system and reduce inflammation during menopause.
- Turmeric contains curcumin, a powerful anti-inflammatory compound that may help alleviate some menopausal symptoms, such as joint pain and hot flashes.
- Ginger and cinnamon also have anti-inflammatory properties and may help improve digestion.
- The black pepper in the smoothie helps enhance the absorption of curcumin from the turmeric.
- Almond milk provides a dairy-free, low-calorie base that is rich in calcium and other essential nutrients.
- The optional honey or maple syrup adds a touch of natural sweetness without the need for excessive added sugars.

This Mango and Turmeric Smoothie is a delicious and nutritious way to incorporate anti-inflammatory ingredients into your menopause diet. Enjoy this vibrant and flavorful smoothie as a healthy snack or breakfast option.

How would you rate this dish?

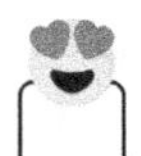 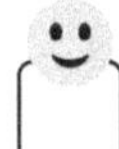 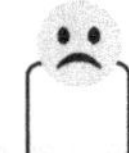 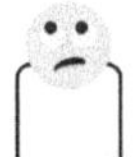 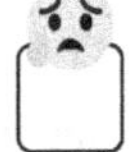

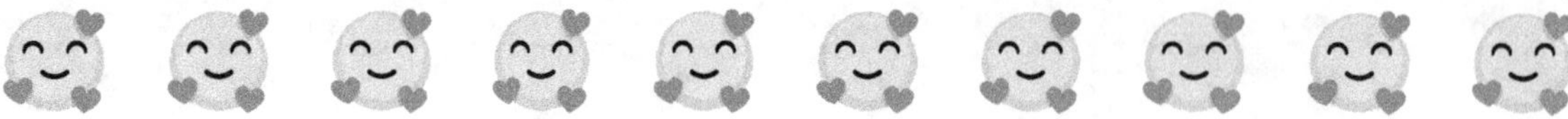

55. Chocolate and Avocado Smoothie

 Prep Time :  Cook Time : Servings :

Write 5 friends with whom you want to share this dish

....

....

....

....

....

Is this dish easy or difficult for you to make?

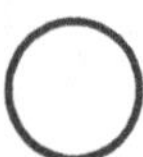 ◯   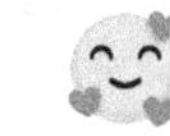 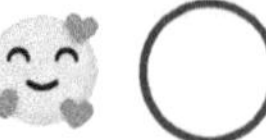 ◯

INGREDIENTS

- 1/2 ripe avocado
- 1 cup unsweetened almond milk
- 2 tablespoons unsweetened cocoa powder
- 1 tablespoon honey (or maple syrup)
- 1 tablespoon ground flaxseed
- 1/2 teaspoon vanilla extract
- Pinch of cinnamon (optional)

1. Add all the ingredients to a high-speed blender.

2. Blend on high speed until the mixture is smooth and creamy, about 1 minute.

3. Taste and adjust sweetener (honey or maple syrup) if desired.

4. Pour the smoothie into a glass and enjoy immediately.

Why this is a great menopause diet option:

- Avocado is a nutrient-dense fruit that provides healthy fats, fiber, and antioxidants to support overall health during menopause.
- Cocoa powder is rich in flavonoids, which have anti-inflammatory properties and may help alleviate some menopausal symptoms.
- Flaxseed is a good source of fiber, omega-3 fatty acids, and lignans, which may help manage menopausal discomforts.
- Honey or maple syrup provide natural sweetness without the use of refined sugars.
- Cinnamon is an anti-inflammatory spice that can also help regulate blood sugar levels.
- The smoothie format makes it easy to consume a nutrient-dense meal or snack.

This Chocolate and Avocado Smoothie is a delicious and satisfying way to incorporate healthy fats, antioxidants, and fiber into your menopause diet. It's a great option for a nutritious breakfast or snack.

How would you rate this dish?

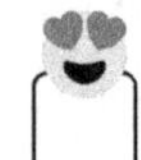 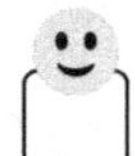  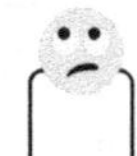 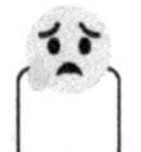

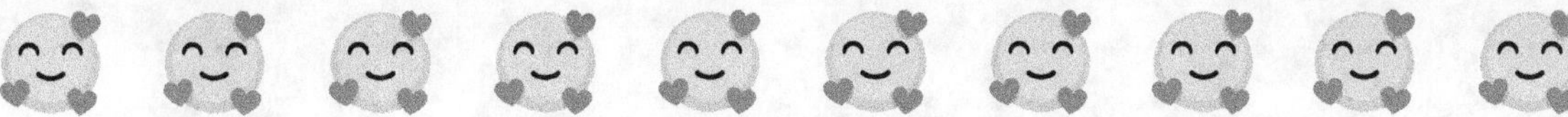

56. Coconut and Pineapple Smoothie

 Prep Time : 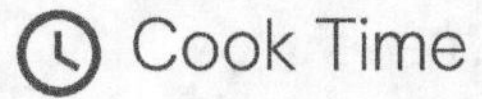 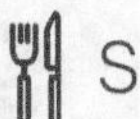 Cook Time : Servings :

Is this dish easy or difficult for you to make?

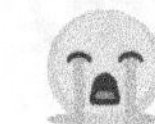 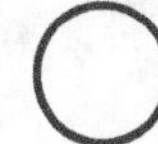 ◯   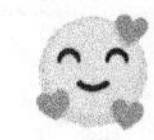 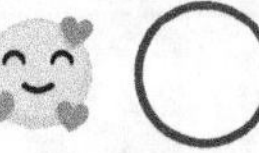 ◯

Write 5 friends with whom you want to share this dish

1. Add all the ingredients to a high-speed blender.

2. Blend on high speed until the mixture is smooth and creamy, about 1 minute.

3. Taste and adjust sweetener (honey) if desired.

4. Pour the smoothie into a glass and enjoy immediately.

Why this smoothie is a great choice:

- Pineapple is a tropical fruit rich in vitamin C, bromelain (an anti-inflammatory enzyme), and fiber.

- Coconut milk provides healthy fats and a creamy, tropical flavor.

- Greek yogurt adds protein to support muscle mass and bone health.

- Honey (if used) provides a natural sweetener.

- Vanilla extract and cinnamon (if used) add warmth and depth of flavor.

This Coconut and Pineapple Smoothie is a refreshing and flavorful way to enjoy a nutrient-dense snack or light meal. The combination of tropical fruits, healthy fats, and protein makes it a satisfying and nourishing choice.

INGREDIENTS

- 1 cup frozen pineapple chunks
- 1/2 cup unsweetened coconut milk (from a can)
- 1/2 cup plain Greek yogurt
- 1 tablespoon honey (optional)
- 1/2 teaspoon vanilla extract
- Pinch of ground cinnamon (optional)

How would you rate this dish?

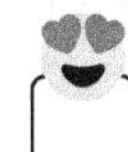 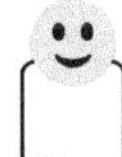 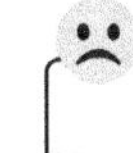 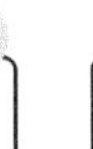 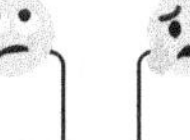 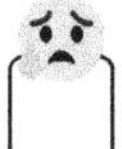

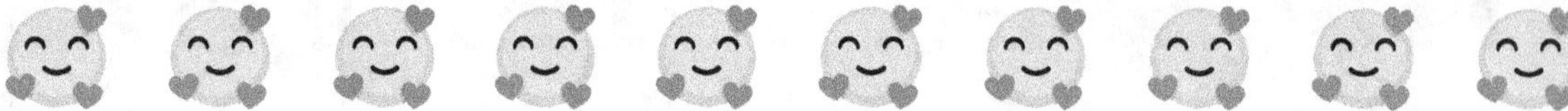

57. Strawberry and Kale Smoothie

 Prep Time :   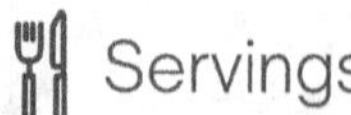 Cook Time :   Servings :

Write 5 friends with whom you want to share this dish

....

....

....

....

....

Is this dish easy or difficult for you to make?

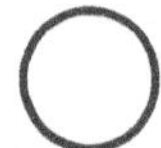 ◯   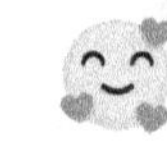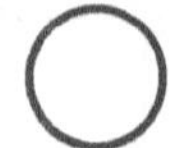 ◯

INGREDIENTS

- 1 cup fresh or frozen strawberries
- 1 cup packed kale leaves, stems removed
- 1 cup unsweetened almond milk (or milk of your choice)
- 1/2 cup plain Greek yogurt
- 1 tablespoon honey (optional)
- 1 teaspoon chia seeds (optional)

1. Add all the ingredients to a high-speed blender.

2. Blend on high speed until the mixture is smooth and creamy, about 1 minute.

3. Taste and adjust sweetener (honey) if desired.

4. Pour the smoothie into a glass and enjoy immediately.

Why this smoothie is a great choice:

- Strawberries are rich in vitamin C, antioxidants, and fiber, which can provide numerous health benefits.

- Kale is a nutrient-dense leafy green packed with vitamins, minerals, and antioxidants.

- Greek yogurt adds protein to support muscle mass and bone health.

- Almond milk is a nutritious dairy-free option that's low in calories and high in vitamins and minerals.

- Honey (if used) provides a natural sweetener.

- Chia seeds are a great source of omega-3 fatty acids, fiber, and protein, which can help promote feelings of fullness.

This Strawberry and Kale Smoothie is a nutrient-dense and refreshing way to start your day or enjoy as a healthy snack. The combination of antioxidants, vitamins, minerals, protein, and fiber makes it a well-balanced and nourishing choice.

How would you rate this dish?

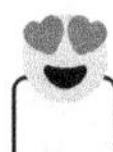 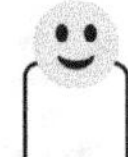 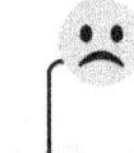 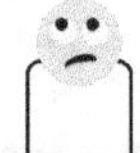 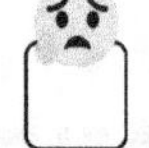

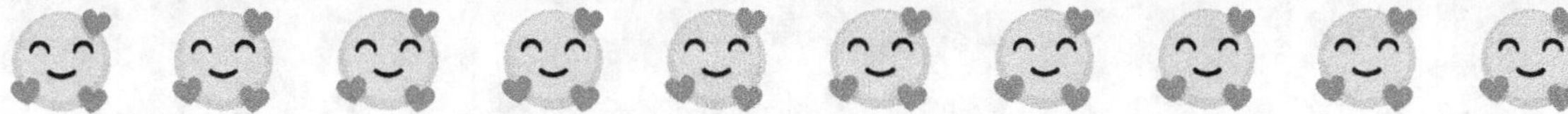

58. Apple and Cinnamon Smoothie

 **Prep Time :**  **Cook Time :** **Servings :**

Let's do that and fill in the time here

Write 5 friends with whom you want to share this dish
....
....
....
....
....

Is this dish easy or difficult for you to make?

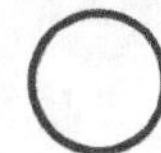 ◯ 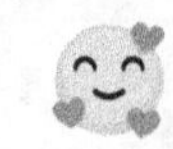 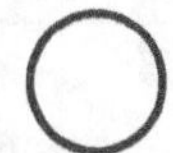 ◯

INGREDIENTS

- 1 medium apple, cored and chopped
- 1 cup unsweetened almond milk
- 1/2 cup plain Greek yogurt
- 1 tablespoon ground flaxseed
- 1 teaspoon ground cinnamon
- 1 teaspoon honey (optional)
- 1/2 teaspoon vanilla extract

1. Add all the ingredients to a high-speed blender.

2. Blend on high speed until the mixture is smooth and creamy, about 1 minute.

3. Taste and adjust sweetener (honey) if desired.

4. Pour the smoothie into a glass and enjoy immediately.

Why this is a great menopause diet option:

- Apples are a good source of fiber, antioxidants, and phytonutrients that can help support overall health during menopause.

- Greek yogurt provides protein to help maintain muscle mass and bone health.

- Flaxseed is a rich source of fiber, omega-3 fatty acids, and lignans, which may help alleviate some menopausal symptoms.

- Cinnamon is an anti-inflammatory spice that can help regulate blood sugar levels and may provide additional benefits.

- Honey (if used) provides a natural sweetener.The smoothie format makes it easy to consume a nutrient-dense meal or snack.

This Apple and Cinnamon Smoothie is a delicious and comforting way to incorporate more fiber, protein, and anti-inflammatory ingredients into your menopause diet. The combination of apples, yogurt, and spices creates a satisfying and nourishing beverage.

How would you rate this dish?

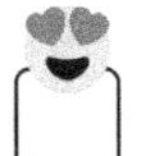  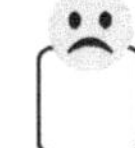 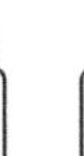 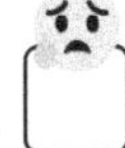

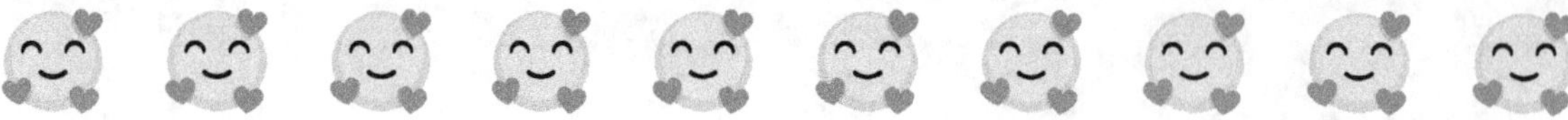

59. Blueberry and Chia Seed Smoothie

 Prep Time : 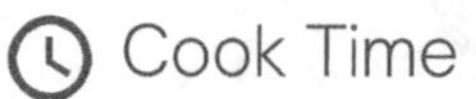 Cook Time :  Servings :

Write 5 friends with whom you want to share this dish ....

Is this dish easy or difficult for you to make?

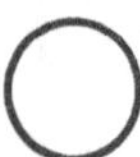 ◯   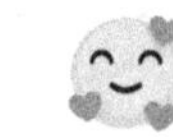 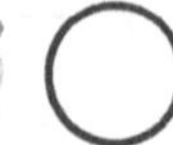 ◯

INGREDIENTS

- 1 cup frozen blueberries
- 1 cup unsweetened almond milk (or milk of your choice)
- 1/2 cup plain Greek yogurt
- 1 tablespoon chia seeds
- 1 tablespoon honey (optional)
- 1/2 teaspoon vanilla extract

1. Add all the ingredients to a high-speed blender.

2. Blend on high speed until the mixture is smooth and creamy, about 1 minute.

3. Taste and adjust sweetener (honey) if desired.

4. Pour the smoothie into a glass and enjoy immediately.

Why this smoothie is a great choice:

- Blueberries are packed with antioxidants, fiber, and vitamins that can provide numerous health benefits.

- Chia seeds are a great source of omega-3 fatty acids, fiber, and protein, which can help promote feelings of fullness.

- Greek yogurt adds protein to support muscle mass and bone health.

- Almond milk is a nutritious dairy-free option that's low in calories and high in vitamins and minerals.

- Honey (if used) provides a natural sweetener.

- Vanilla extract adds a delicious flavor.

This Blueberry and Chia Seed Smoothie is a nutrient-dense and satisfying way to start your day or enjoy as a healthy snack. The combination of antioxidants, healthy fats, protein, and fiber makes it a well-balanced and nourishing choice.

How would you rate this dish?

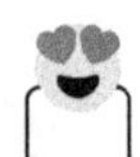 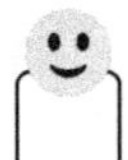 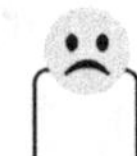 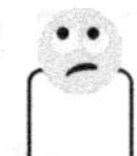 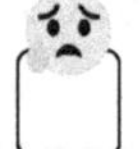

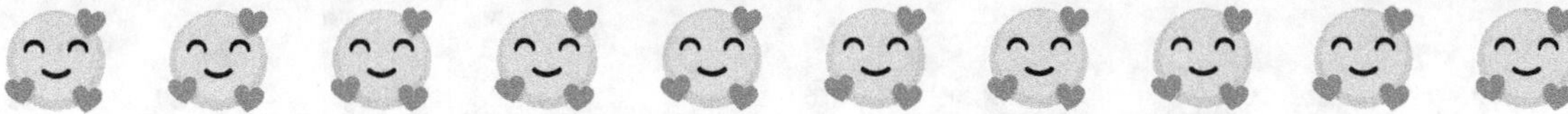

60. Peach and Ginger Smoothie

 Prep Time : 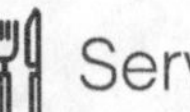 Cook Time : 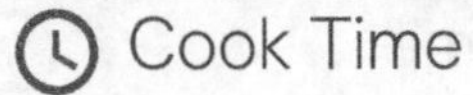 Servings :

Write 5 friends with whom you want to share this dish

....
....
....
....
....

INGREDIENTS

- 1 cup frozen peach slices
- 1 cup unsweetened almond milk (or milk of your choice)
- 1/2 cup plain Greek yogurt
- 1 tablespoon honey (optional)
- 1 teaspoon freshly grated ginger
- 1/2 teaspoon vanilla extract

Is this dish easy or difficult for you to make?

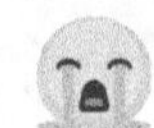 ◯   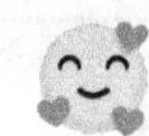 ◯

1. Add all the ingredients to a high-speed blender.

2. Blend on high speed until the mixture is smooth and creamy, about 1 minute.

3. Taste and adjust sweetener (honey) if desired.

4. Pour the smoothie into a glass and enjoy immediately.

Why this smoothie is a great choice:

- Peaches are a juicy, seasonal fruit that are rich in vitamins, minerals, and antioxidants.

- Ginger is an anti-inflammatory ingredient that can help soothe the digestive system and provide a subtle spicy kick.

- Greek yogurt adds protein to support muscle mass and bone health.

- Almond milk is a nutritious dairy-free option that's low in calories and high in vitamins and minerals.

- Honey (if used) provides a natural sweetener.

- Vanilla extract adds a delicious flavor.

This Peach and Ginger Smoothie is a refreshing and nourishing way to start your day or enjoy as a healthy snack. The combination of sweet peaches, tangy yogurt, and spicy ginger creates a delightful and satisfying beverage.

How would you rate this dish?

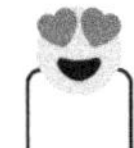   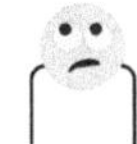 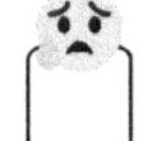

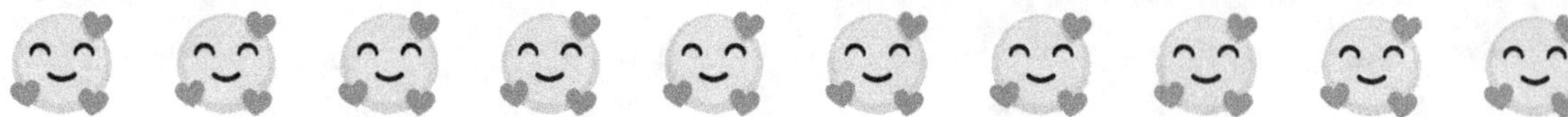

61. Chicken and Vegetable Soup

 Prep Time :  Cook Time : Servings :

Write 5 friends with whom you want to share this dish

Is this dish easy or difficult for you to make?

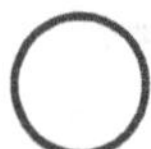 ◯ 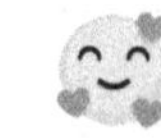 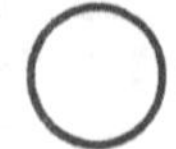 ◯

INGREDIENTS

- 1 tablespoon olive oil
- 1 onion, diced
- 3 cloves garlic, minced
- 2 carrots, peeled and sliced
- 2 celery stalks, sliced
- 1 cup chopped broccoli florets
- 1 cup chopped cauliflower florets
- 4 cups low-sodium chicken broth
- 2 cups shredded cooked chicken breast
- 1 teaspoon dried thyme
- 1 bay leaf
- Salt and black pepper to taste
- 2 cups baby spinach leaves

1. In a large pot or Dutch oven, heat the olive oil over medium heat. Add the diced onion and sauté for 5 minutes until translucent.

2. Add the minced garlic and sauté for an additional 1-2 minutes until fragrant.

3. Stir in the sliced carrots, celery, broccoli, and cauliflower. Pour in the chicken broth and add the shredded cooked chicken, dried thyme, and bay leaf.

4. Bring the soup to a simmer and let it cook for 15-20 minutes, or until the vegetables are tender.

5. Remove the bay leaf. Season the soup with salt and black pepper to taste.

6. Just before serving, stir in the baby spinach leaves and let them wilt for 1-2 minutes.

7. Ladle the hot chicken and vegetable soup into bowls and serve.

Why this is a great menopause diet option:

- The vegetables provide a variety of vitamins, minerals, and antioxidants to support overall health during menopause.
- Chicken is a lean protein source that can help maintain muscle mass.
- Spinach is a nutrient-dense green that's rich in calcium, which is important for bone health.
- The broth-based soup format is easy to digest and hydrating.

How would you rate this dish?

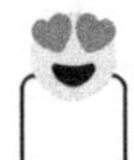 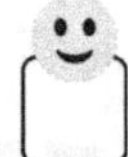 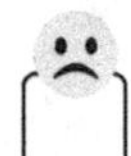 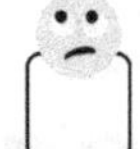 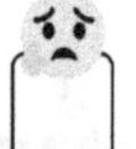

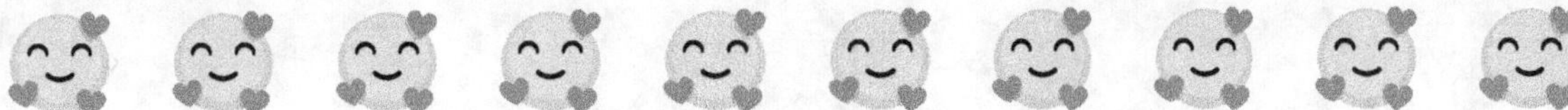

62. Lentil and Spinach Soup

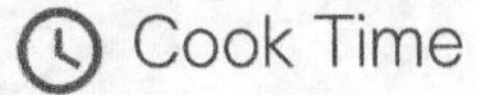 Prep Time :    Cook Time :   Servings :

Write 5 friends with whom you want to share this dish

....

....

....

....

....

Is this dish easy or difficult for you to make?

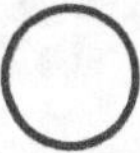 ◯   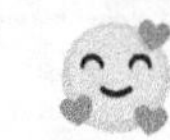 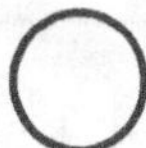 ◯

INGREDIENTS

- 1 tablespoon olive oil
- 1 onion, diced
- 3 cloves garlic, minced
- 1 cup dried brown or green lentils, rinsed
- 4 cups low-sodium vegetable or chicken broth
- 1 (14.5 oz) can diced tomatoes
- 1 teaspoon ground cumin
- 1 teaspoon dried oregano
- 1/4 teaspoon red pepper flakes (optional)
- Salt and black pepper to taste
- 2 cups fresh spinach leaves, chopped

1. In a large pot or Dutch oven, heat the olive oil over medium heat. Add the diced onion and sauté for 5-7 minutes until translucent.

2. Add the minced garlic and sauté for an additional 1-2 minutes until fragrant.

3. Stir in the rinsed lentils, vegetable or chicken broth, diced tomatoes, cumin, oregano, and red pepper flakes (if using). Season with salt and black pepper to taste.

4. Bring the soup to a boil, then reduce the heat and let it simmer for 20-25 minutes, or until the lentils are tender.

5. Just before serving, stir in the chopped fresh spinach leaves and let them wilt for 1-2 minutes. Ladle the hot lentil and spinach soup into bowls and serve.

Why this is a great menopause diet option:

- Lentils are a plant-based protein source that can help maintain muscle mass and provide sustained energy.
- Spinach is a nutrient-dense green that's rich in vitamins, minerals, and antioxidants to support overall health during menopause.
- The combination of protein, fiber, and complex carbohydrates from the lentils and vegetables can help regulate blood sugar levels.
- Cumin and oregano are anti-inflammatory spices that may help alleviate some menopausal symptoms.
- The broth-based soup format is easy to digest and hydrating

How would you rate this dish?

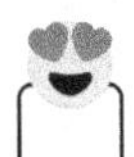 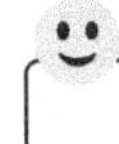  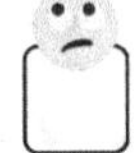 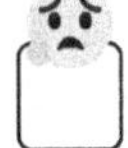

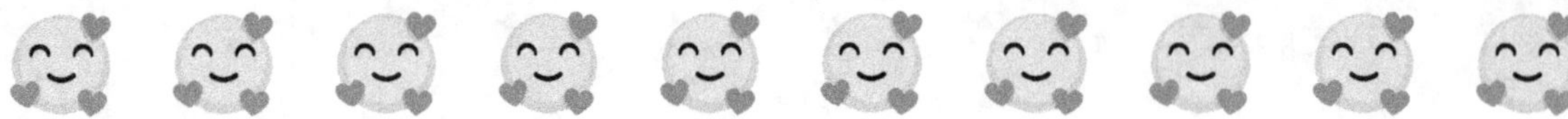

63. Tomato and Basil Soup

 Prep Time :   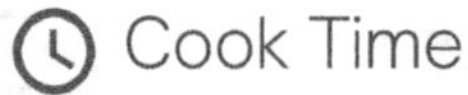 Cook Time :   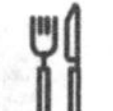 Servings :

Is this dish easy or difficult for you to make?

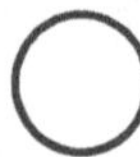 ◯   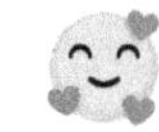 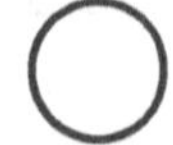 ◯

Write 5 friends with whom you want to share this dish ....

INGREDIENTS

- 2 tablespoons olive oil
- 1 onion, diced
- 3 cloves garlic, minced
- 1 (28 oz) can diced tomatoes
- 2 cups low-sodium vegetable or chicken broth
- 1/4 cup fresh basil leaves, chopped
- 1 teaspoon dried oregano
- 1/4 teaspoon red pepper flakes (optional)
- Salt and black pepper to taste
- 1/2 cup plain Greek yogurt (for serving)

1. In a large saucepan or Dutch oven, heat the olive oil over medium heat. Add the diced onion and sauté for 5-7 minutes until translucent.

2. Add the minced garlic and sauté for an additional 1-2 minutes until fragrant.

3. Pour in the canned diced tomatoes and the vegetable or chicken broth. Bring the mixture to a simmer.

4. Stir in the chopped fresh basil, dried oregano, and red pepper flakes (if using). Season with salt and black pepper to taste.

5. Reduce the heat to low and let the soup simmer for 15-20 minutes, allowing the flavors to meld.

6. Using an immersion blender or regular blender, carefully blend the soup until smooth and creamy.

7. Serve the tomato and basil soup warm, topped with a dollop of plain Greek yogurt.

Why this is a great menopause diet option:

- Tomatoes are rich in lycopene, an antioxidant that may help reduce the risk of certain cancers and heart disease.
- Basil is an anti-inflammatory herb that can help alleviate some menopausal symptoms.
- Greek yogurt provides protein to support muscle mass and bone health.
- The soup format is a comforting and easy-to-digest option.

How would you rate this dish?

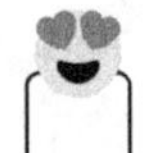   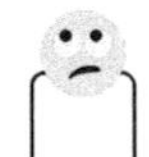 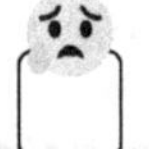

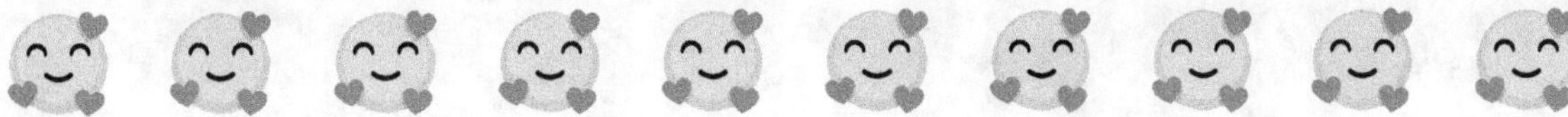

64. Butternut Squash Soup

 Prep Time :  Cook Time : Servings :

Is this dish easy or difficult for you to make?

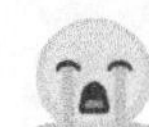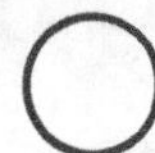 ◯   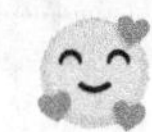 ◯

Write 5 friends with whom you want to share this dish

....

....

....

....

....

INGREDIENTS

- 1 medium butternut squash, peeled, seeded, and cubed (about 4 cups)
- 1 onion, diced
- 2 cloves garlic, minced
- 4 cups low-sodium vegetable or chicken broth
- 1 cup unsweetened almond milk (or milk of your choice)
- 1 teaspoon ground cumin
- 1/2 teaspoon ground cinnamon
- 1/4 teaspoon ground nutmeg
- Salt and black pepper to taste
- Chopped fresh parsley or chives for garnish (optional)

1. In a large pot or Dutch oven, sauté the diced onion in a drizzle of olive oil over medium heat for 5-7 minutes until translucent.

2. Add the minced garlic and sauté for an additional 1-2 minutes until fragrant.

3. Add the cubed butternut squash, vegetable or chicken broth, almond milk, cumin, cinnamon, and nutmeg. Season with salt and black pepper to taste.

4. Bring the mixture to a boil, then reduce the heat and let it simmer for 20-25 minutes, or until the squash is very soft.

5. Using an immersion blender or regular blender, carefully blend the soup until smooth and creamy.

6. Return the blended soup to the pot and heat through, adjusting seasoning if needed.

7. Ladle the butternut squash soup into bowls and garnish with chopped fresh parsley or chives, if desired.

Serve the soup warm, with crusty bread or a side salad for a complete and nourishing meal.

This Butternut Squash Soup is a comforting, flavorful, and nutrient-dense option that's perfect for a chilly day. The combination of sweet squash, warming spices, and creamy texture makes it a delightful and satisfying soup.

How would you rate this dish?

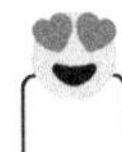 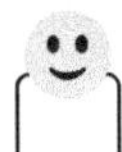  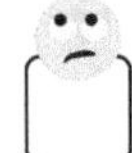 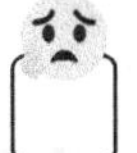

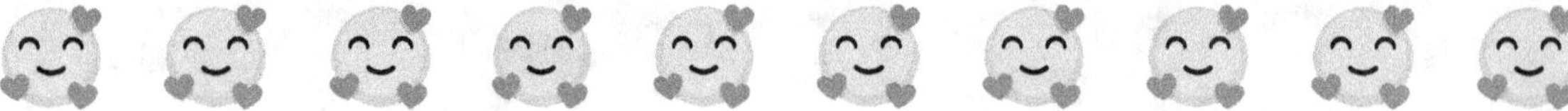

65. Miso Soup with Tofu and Seaweed

 Prep Time : 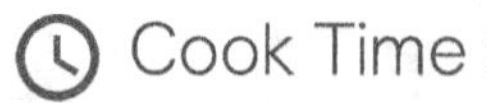 Cook Time : 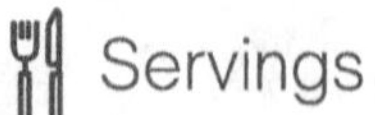 Servings :

Write 5 friends with whom you want to share this dish

....
....
....
....
....

Is this dish easy or difficult for you to make?

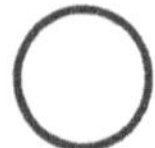 ◯ 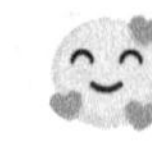 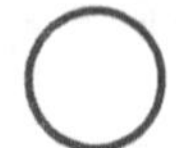 ◯

INGREDIENTS

- 4 cups low-sodium vegetable or chicken broth
- 2 tablespoons white or yellow miso paste
- 1 block (14 oz) firm or extra-firm tofu, cubed
- 1 cup thinly sliced shiitake mushrooms
- 1/2 cup thinly sliced green onions
- 2 tablespoons dried wakame seaweed (or other seaweed)
- 1 teaspoon grated fresh ginger
- 1 tablespoon low-sodium soy sauce (optional)

1. In a medium saucepan, bring the broth to a gentle simmer over medium heat.

2. In a small bowl, whisk the miso paste with a few tablespoons of the hot broth until smooth. Pour the miso mixture back into the saucepan, stirring to combine.

3. Add the cubed tofu, sliced shiitake mushrooms, green onions, dried wakame seaweed, and grated ginger to the simmering broth.

4. Cook for 5-7 minutes, allowing the flavors to meld.

5. Taste and stir in the soy sauce if desired.

6. Ladle the miso soup into bowls and serve hot.

Why this is a great menopause diet option:

- Miso is a fermented soy product that contains probiotics, which can support gut health.
- Tofu is a plant-based protein source that can help maintain muscle mass.
- Shiitake mushrooms and wakame seaweed are rich in vitamins, minerals, and antioxidants.
- Ginger has anti-inflammatory properties that may help alleviate some menopausal symptoms.
- The broth-based soup format is easy to digest and hydrating.

This Miso Soup with Tofu and Seaweed is a nourishing, flavorful, and menopause-friendly meal that can be enjoyed as a light lunch or dinner.

How would you rate this dish?

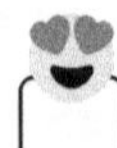 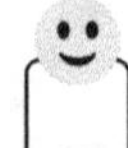 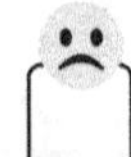 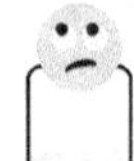 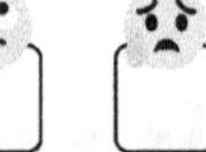

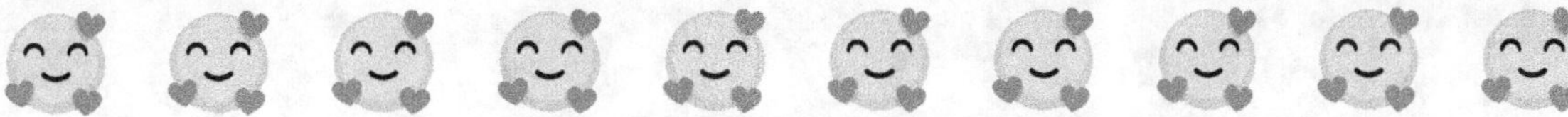

66. Vegetable Minestrone Soup

 Prep Time :

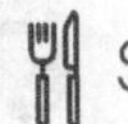 Cook Time :

Servings :

Write 5 friends with whom you want to share this dish

....

....

....

....

....

Is this dish easy or difficult for you to make?

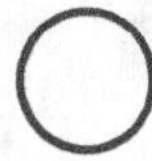 ◯   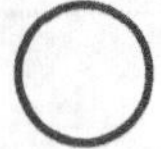 ◯

INGREDIENTS

- 2 tablespoons olive oil
- 1 onion, diced
- 3 cloves garlic, minced
- 2 carrots, peeled and diced
- 2 stalks celery, diced
- 1 zucchini, diced
- 1 (15 oz) can diced tomatoes
- 4 cups low-sodium vegetable or chicken broth
- 1 (15 oz) can kidney beans, rinsed and drained
- 1 cup small pasta (like ditalini or elbow macaroni)
- 2 cups chopped kale or spinach
- 1 teaspoon dried oregano
- 1/2 teaspoon dried basil
- Salt and pepper to taste
- Grated Parmesan cheese for serving (optional)

1. In a large pot, heat the olive oil over medium heat. Add the onion and sauté for 5 minutes until translucent.

2. Add the garlic, carrots, celery, and zucchini. Cook for 5 more minutes, stirring occasionally.

3. Pour in the diced tomatoes and their juices, along with the broth. Bring to a simmer.

4. Add the kidney beans, pasta, kale/spinach, oregano, and basil. Season with salt and pepper.

5. Simmer for 15-20 minutes, until the pasta is tender.

6. Ladle the soup into bowls and top with a sprinkle of Parmesan cheese if desired.

This hearty vegetable minestrone is packed with fiber, vitamins, and minerals - all important for supporting women's health during menopause. The tomatoes provide lycopene, while the beans and greens offer phytoestrogens. Enjoy!

How would you rate this dish?

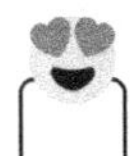 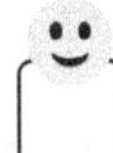 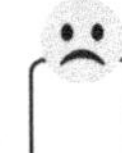 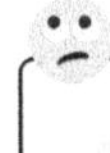 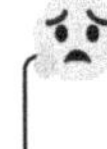

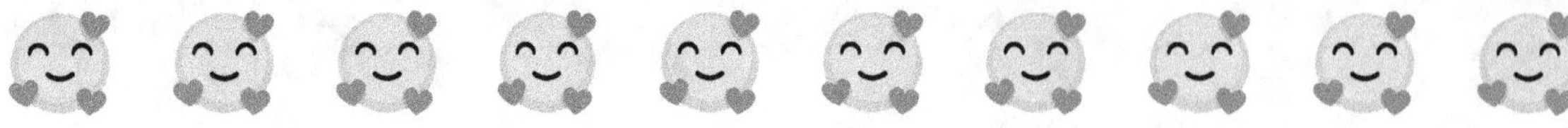

67. Pumpkin Soup with Coconut Milk

 Prep Time :  Cook Time : Servings :

Is this dish easy or difficult for you to make?

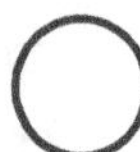 ◯  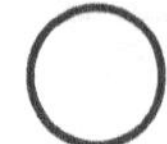 ◯

Write 5 friends with whom you want to share this dish

....
....
....
....
....

INGREDIENTS

- 1 small sugar pumpkin or 2 cups canned pumpkin puree
- 1 tablespoon olive oil
- 1 onion, diced
- 3 cloves garlic, minced
- 1 teaspoon ground cumin
- 1 teaspoon ground coriander
- 1/4 teaspoon cayenne pepper (or to taste)
- 1 (13.5 oz) can coconut milk
- 2 cups vegetable or chicken broth
- Salt and pepper to taste
- Chopped cilantro for garnish

1. If using a whole pumpkin, cut it in half, scoop out the seeds, and roast at 400°F for 45-60 minutes until very soft. Scoop out the flesh and puree until smooth.

2. In a large pot, heat the olive oil over medium heat. Add the onion and sauté for 5 minutes until translucent. Add the garlic, cumin, coriander, and cayenne. Cook for 1 minute until fragrant.

3. Pour in the coconut milk and broth. Add the pumpkin puree and stir to combine. Bring to a simmer and cook for 10-15 minutes, stirring occasionally, until heated through.

4. Season with salt and pepper to taste.

5. Ladle the soup into bowls and garnish with chopped cilantro.

Enjoy this creamy, flavorful pumpkin soup! The coconut milk adds a lovely richness.

How would you rate this dish?

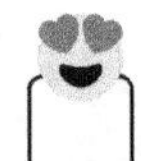 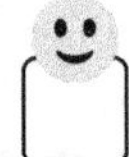 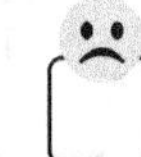 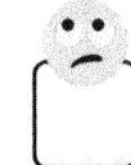 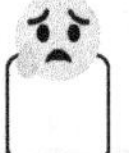

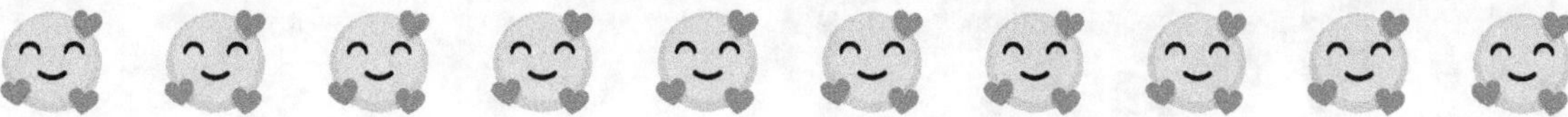

68. Broccoli and Cheddar Soup

 Prep Time : 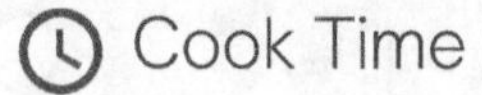  Cook Time : Servings :

Is this dish easy or difficult for you to make?

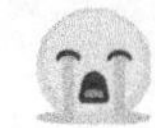 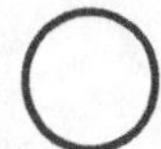 ◯   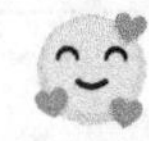 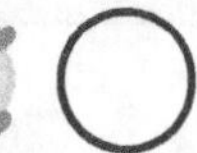 ◯

Write 5 friends with whom you want to share this dish

....

....

....

....

....

INGREDIENTS

- 2 tablespoons olive oil
- 1 onion, diced
- 3 cloves garlic, minced
- 4 cups low-sodium chicken or vegetable broth
- 4 cups chopped broccoli florets
- 1 cup shredded low-fat cheddar cheese
- 1/4 cup plain Greek yogurt
- 1 teaspoon Dijon mustard
- 1/4 teaspoon ground nutmeg
- Salt and black pepper to taste

1. In a large pot or Dutch oven, heat the olive oil over medium heat. Add the diced onion and sauté for 5-7 minutes until translucent.

2. Add the minced garlic and sauté for an additional 1-2 minutes until fragrant.

3. Pour in the chicken or vegetable broth and add the chopped broccoli florets. Bring the mixture to a simmer and cook for 10-15 minutes, or until the broccoli is tender.

4. Using an immersion blender or regular blender, carefully blend the soup until smooth and creamy.

5. Return the blended soup to the pot and stir in the shredded low-fat cheddar cheese, plain Greek yogurt, Dijon mustard, and ground nutmeg.

6. Season with salt and black pepper to taste.

7. Heat the soup through, stirring occasionally, until the cheese is melted and the soup is hot.

8. Ladle the broccoli and cheddar soup into bowls and serve.

This Broccoli and Cheddar Soup is a comforting, nourishing, and menopause-friendly meal that can be enjoyed for lunch or dinner.

How would you rate this dish?

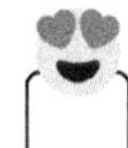 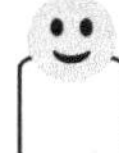 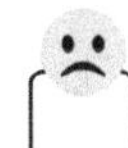 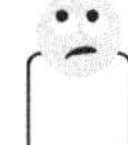 

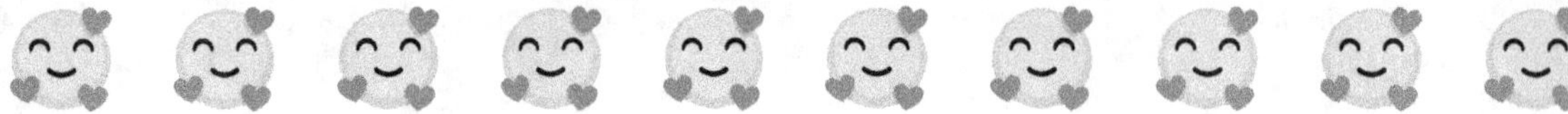

69. Carrot and Ginger Soup

 Prep Time :   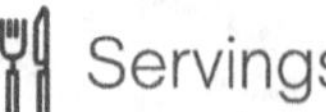 Cook Time :   Servings :

Is this dish easy or difficult for you to make?

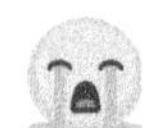 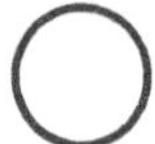 ◯     ◯

Write 5 friends with whom you want to share this dish

....

....

....

....

....

INGREDIENTS

- 2 tablespoons olive oil
- 1 onion, diced
- 3 cloves garlic, minced
- 1 tablespoon grated fresh ginger
- 1 lb carrots, peeled and sliced
- 4 cups low-sodium vegetable or chicken broth
- 1 cup unsweetened almond milk
- 1 teaspoon ground cumin
- 1/4 teaspoon cayenne pepper (optional)
- Salt and pepper to taste
- Chopped cilantro for garnish (optional)

1. In a large pot, heat the olive oil over medium heat. Add the onion and sauté for 5 minutes until translucent.

2. Add the garlic and ginger. Cook for 1 minute, stirring constantly, until fragrant.

3. Add the sliced carrots and broth. Bring to a simmer and cook for 20-25 minutes, until the carrots are very soft.

4. Remove the pot from heat and use an immersion blender to puree the soup until smooth. Alternatively, you can transfer the soup to a regular blender in batches and blend until creamy.

5. Stir in the almond milk, cumin, and cayenne (if using). Season with salt and pepper to taste.

6. Return the soup to low heat and cook for 5 more minutes, stirring occasionally, until heated through.

7. Ladle the soup into bowls and garnish with chopped cilantro if desired.

This carrot and ginger soup is a wonderful option for a menopause-friendly diet. Carrots are high in beta-carotene, which can help reduce hot flashes. Ginger has anti-inflammatory properties that may ease joint pain. The almond milk makes it dairy-free. Enjoy this nourishing and flavorful soup!

How would you rate this dish?

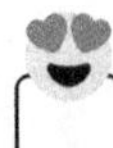 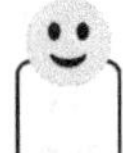 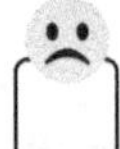 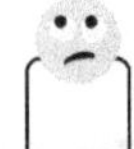 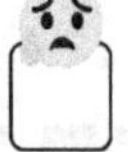

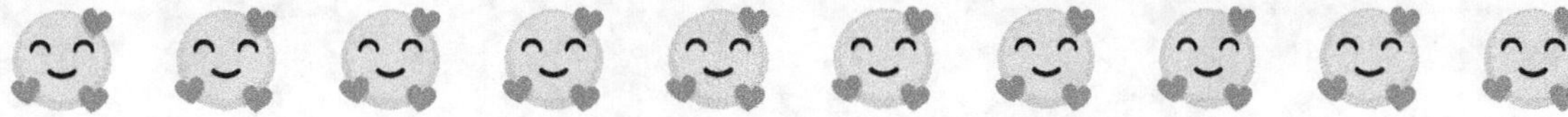

70. Cauliflower Soup with Garlic

 Prep Time :   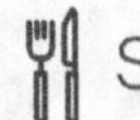 Cook Time :   Servings :

Write 5 friends with whom you want to share this dish

....

....

....

....

....

....

Is this dish easy or difficult for you to make?

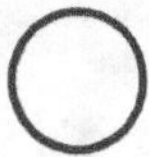 ◯   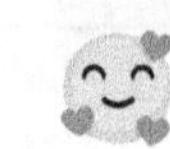 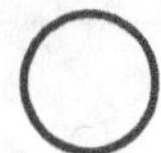 ◯

INGREDIENTS

- 1 head of cauliflower, cut into florets
- 2 tablespoons olive oil
- 1 onion, diced
- 4 cloves garlic, minced
- 4 cups low-sodium vegetable or chicken broth
- 1 cup unsweetened almond milk
- 1 teaspoon dried thyme
- Salt and pepper to taste
- Chopped parsley for garnish (optional)

1. In a large pot, bring a few inches of water to a boil. Add the cauliflower florets and steam for 10-12 minutes until very tender. Drain and set aside.

2. In the same pot, heat the olive oil over medium heat. Add the onion and sauté for 5 minutes until translucent.

3. Add the garlic and cook for 1 minute more, until fragrant.

4. Pour in the broth and almond milk. Add the steamed cauliflower and thyme. Season with salt and pepper.

5. Use an immersion blender to puree the soup until smooth and creamy. Alternatively, you can transfer the soup to a regular blender in batches and blend until smooth.

6. Return the soup to the pot and heat through. Taste and adjust seasonings as needed.

7. Ladle the soup into bowls and garnish with chopped parsley if desired.

This creamy cauliflower soup is an excellent option for a menopause-friendly diet. Cauliflower is high in fiber, folate, and antioxidants, while the garlic provides anti-inflammatory benefits. The almond milk makes it dairy-free. Enjoy this comforting and nutritious soup!

How would you rate this dish?

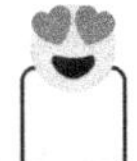   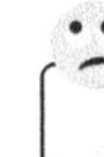  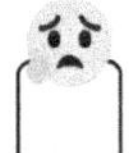

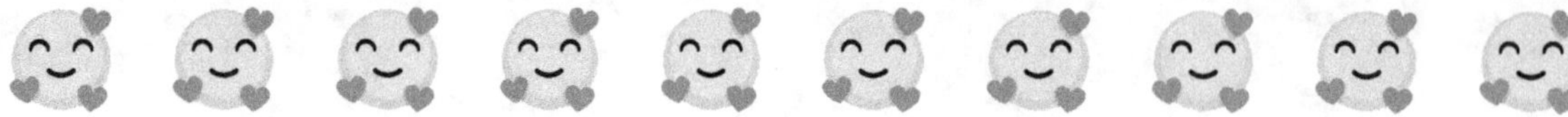

71. Kale and Quinoa Salad with Lemon Dressing

 *Let's do that and fill in the time here*

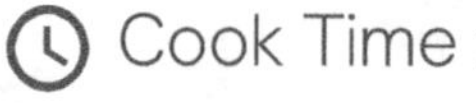 Prep Time :  Cook Time : Servings :

Write 5 friends with whom you want to share this dish

....

....

....

....

....

INGREDIENTS

Salad:
- 4 cups chopped kale, stems removed
- 1 cup cooked quinoa, cooled
- 1/2 cup diced cucumber
- 1/2 cup diced bell pepper
- 1/4 cup crumbled feta cheese (optional)
- 2 tablespoons toasted sliced almonds

Lemon Dressing:
- 2 tablespoons fresh lemon juice
- 1 tablespoon olive oil
- 1 teaspoon Dijon mustard
- 1 teaspoon honey
- 1/4 teaspoon salt
- 1/8 teaspoon black pepper

Is this dish easy or difficult for you to make?

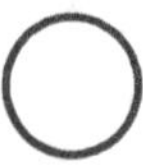 ◯   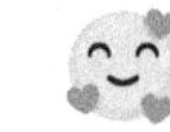 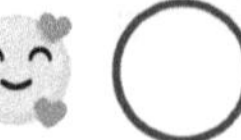 ◯

1. In a large bowl, combine the chopped kale, cooked quinoa, diced cucumber, diced bell pepper, crumbled feta (if using), and toasted sliced almonds.

2. In a small bowl, whisk together the lemon juice, olive oil, Dijon mustard, honey, salt, and black pepper to make the dressing.

3. Pour the lemon dressing over the salad and toss gently to coat the ingredients evenly.

4. Let the salad sit for 5-10 minutes to allow the kale to soften slightly before serving.

Why this is a great menopause diet option:

- Kale is a nutrient-dense leafy green that's rich in vitamins, minerals, and antioxidants to support overall health during menopause.
- Quinoa is a high-protein, gluten-free grain that can help maintain muscle mass and energy levels.
- Vegetables like cucumber and bell pepper provide additional vitamins, minerals, and fiber.
- Feta cheese (if used) is a good source of calcium, which is important for bone health.
- Almonds are a healthy source of protein, fiber, and beneficial fats.
- The lemon dressing provides a refreshing, tangy flavor and contains anti-inflammatory properties.

This Kale and Quinoa Salad with Lemon Dressing is a nourishing, balanced, and delicious option for a menopause-friendly meal or side dish.

How would you rate this dish?

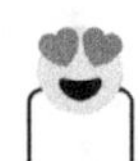 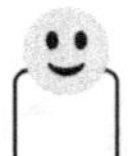  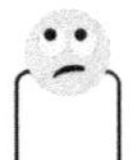 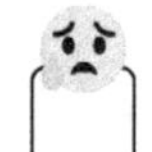

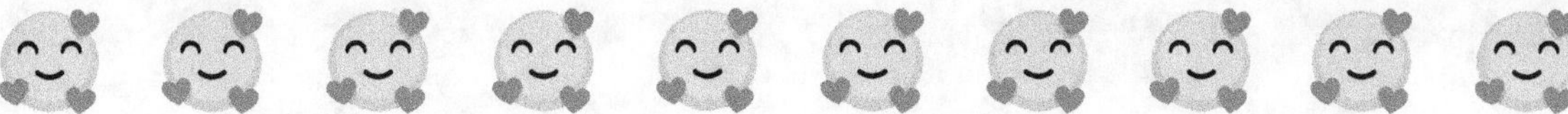

72. Spinach and Feta Salad with Olives

 Prep Time : 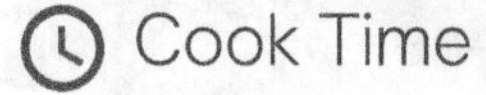 Cook Time : 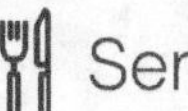 Servings :

Is this dish easy or difficult for you to make?

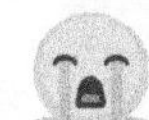 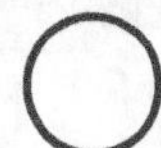 ◯   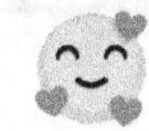 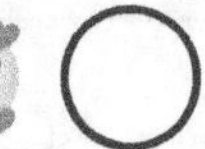 ◯

Write 5 friends with whom you want to share this dish

....

....

....

....

....

INGREDIENTS

- 5 oz baby spinach leaves
- 1/2 cup crumbled feta cheese
- 1/4 cup pitted kalamata olives, halved
- 2 tablespoons toasted pine nuts
- 2 tablespoons extra virgin olive oil
- 1 tablespoon balsamic vinegar
- 1 teaspoon Dijon mustard
- 1 teaspoon honey
- Salt and pepper to taste

1. In a large salad bowl, combine the baby spinach, crumbled feta, halved olives, and toasted pine nuts.

2. In a small bowl, whisk together the olive oil, balsamic vinegar, Dijon mustard, and honey. Season with salt and pepper.

3. Drizzle the dressing over the salad and toss gently to coat.

4. Serve the spinach and feta salad immediately.

This spinach salad is an excellent choice for a menopause-friendly diet. Spinach is packed with vitamins, minerals, and antioxidants that can help support women's health during this transition. The feta cheese provides calcium, while the olives offer healthy fats.

The balsamic vinaigrette dressing is light and tangy, complementing the flavors of the salad. The toasted pine nuts add a nice crunch.

This salad can be enjoyed as a main course or a side dish. It's a nutritious and delicious way to incorporate more plant-based foods into your diet.

How would you rate this dish?

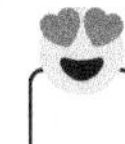 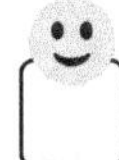  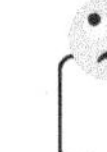 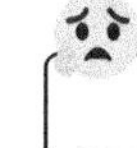

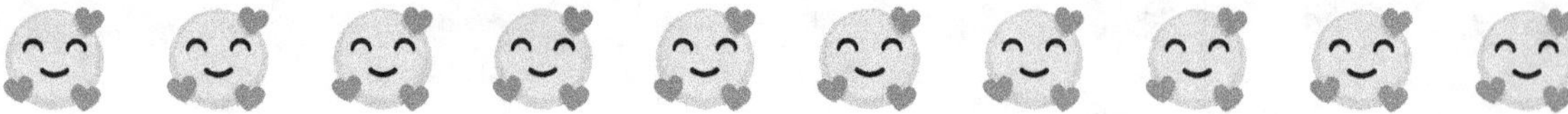

73. Cabbage and Carrot Slaw with Yogurt Dressing

 Prep Time :  Cook Time : Servings :

Write 5 friends with whom you want to share this dish

....

....

....

....

....

INGREDIENTS

- 1/2 head green cabbage, shredded
- 2 carrots, grated
- 1/2 red onion, thinly sliced
- 1 cup plain Greek yogurt
- 2 tablespoons apple cider vinegar
- 1 tablespoon honey
- 1 teaspoon Dijon mustard
- 1/4 teaspoon ground cumin
- Salt and pepper to taste
- Chopped fresh parsley for garnish (optional)

Is this dish easy or difficult for you to make?

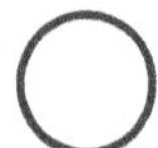 ◯   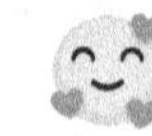 ◯

1. In a large bowl, combine the shredded cabbage, grated carrots, and sliced red onion.

2. In a small bowl, whisk together the Greek yogurt, apple cider vinegar, honey, Dijon mustard, and cumin. Season with salt and pepper.

3. Pour the yogurt dressing over the cabbage and carrot mixture and toss to coat evenly.

4. Cover and refrigerate the slaw for at least 30 minutes to allow the flavors to meld.

5. Just before serving, give the slaw another gentle toss.

6. Transfer to a serving bowl and garnish with chopped fresh parsley if desired.

This cabbage and carrot slaw is a great option for a menopause-friendly diet. Cabbage is high in fiber and antioxidants, while carrots provide beta-carotene. The yogurt dressing adds protein and probiotics. The apple cider vinegar may help regulate blood sugar levels.

This slaw is crunchy, tangy, and lightly sweet - a perfect side dish or topping for grilled meats or fish. Enjoy!

How would you rate this dish?

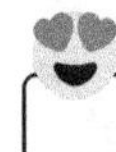 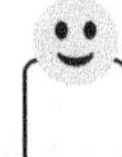 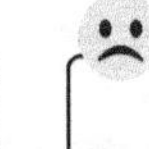 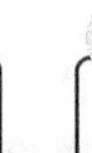 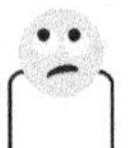 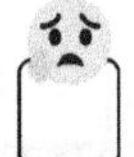

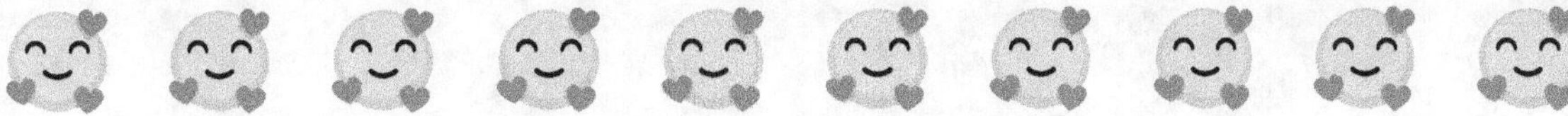

74. Roasted Sweet Potato Salad with Arugula

 Prep Time :

 Cook Time :   Servings :

Write 5 friends with whom you want to share this dish

....

....

....

....

....

Is this dish easy or difficult for you to make?

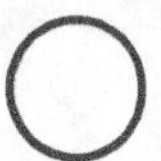 ◯   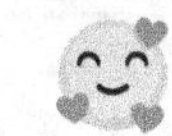 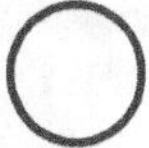 ◯

INGREDIENTS

- 3 medium sweet potatoes, peeled and cubed
- 2 tablespoons olive oil
- Salt and pepper to taste
- 5 oz baby arugula
- 1/4 cup crumbled feta cheese
- 2 tablespoons toasted pumpkin seeds
- 2 tablespoons balsamic vinegar
- 1 tablespoon Dijon mustard
- 1 tablespoon honey

1. Preheat the oven to 400°F. Toss the cubed sweet potatoes with the olive oil and season with salt and pepper. Spread in a single layer on a baking sheet.

2. Roast the sweet potatoes for 20-25 minutes, flipping halfway, until tender and lightly browned. Allow to cool slightly.

3. In a large salad bowl, combine the roasted sweet potatoes, baby arugula, crumbled feta, and toasted pumpkin seeds.

4. In a small bowl, whisk together the balsamic vinegar, Dijon mustard, and honey. Season with salt and pepper.

5. Drizzle the balsamic dressing over the salad and toss gently to coat.

6. Serve the roasted sweet potato salad immediately.

This salad is an excellent choice for a menopause-friendly diet. Sweet potatoes are high in beta-carotene, which can help reduce hot flashes. Arugula is packed with antioxidants and fiber. The feta cheese provides calcium, while the pumpkin seeds offer healthy fats and minerals.

The balsamic vinaigrette dressing adds a tangy, slightly sweet flavor that complements the other ingredients. This salad is a nutritious and delicious way to incorporate more plant-based foods into your diet.

How would you rate this dish?

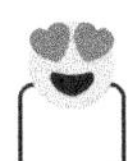 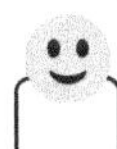  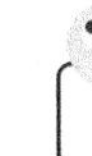 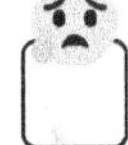

75. Chickpea and Cucumber Salad

 *Let's do that and fill in the time here* 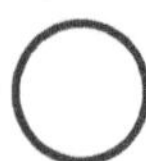 Prep Time :   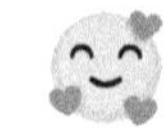 Cook Time :   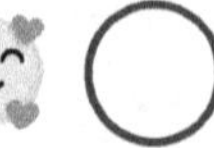 Servings :

Write 5 friends with whom you want to share this dish

....
....
....
....
....

Is this dish easy or difficult for you to make?

 ◯   ◯

INGREDIENTS

- 1 (15 oz) can chickpeas, rinsed and drained
- 1 English cucumber, diced
- 1/2 red onion, thinly sliced
- 1/4 cup chopped fresh parsley
- 2 tablespoons extra virgin olive oil
- 2 tablespoons lemon juice
- 1 teaspoon Dijon mustard
- 1/2 teaspoon ground cumin
- Salt and pepper to taste

1. In a large bowl, combine the chickpeas, cucumber, red onion, and parsley.

2. In a small bowl, whisk together the olive oil, lemon juice, Dijon mustard, and cumin. Season with salt and pepper.

3. Pour the dressing over the chickpea and vegetable mixture and toss gently to coat.

4. Let the salad sit for 10-15 minutes to allow the flavors to meld.

5. Serve chilled or at room temperature.

This chickpea and cucumber salad is an excellent option for a menopause-friendly diet. Chickpeas are a great source of plant-based protein, fiber, and complex carbohydrates. Cucumbers are hydrating and contain antioxidants that may help reduce inflammation. The lemon juice and Dijon provide a tangy dressing that complements the vegetables.

This salad can be enjoyed on its own or served over a bed of greens. It's a refreshing and nutritious side dish or light main course. Enjoy!

How would you rate this dish?

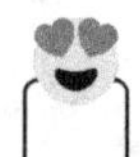 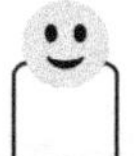 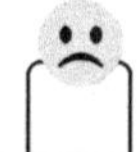 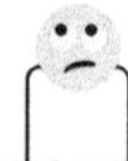 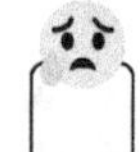

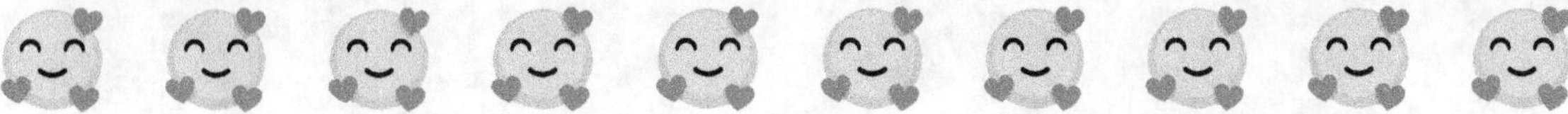

76. Farro Salad with Tomatoes and Basil

 *Let's do that and fill in the time here*

Prep Time :

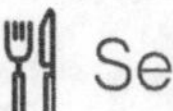 Cook Time :

Servings :

Write 5 friends with whom you want to share this dish

....

....

....

....

....

Is this dish easy or difficult for you to make?

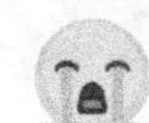  ◯   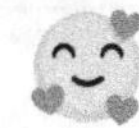 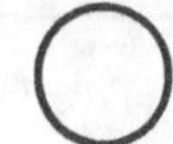 ◯

INGREDIENTS

- 1 cup uncooked farro
- 2 cups cherry or grape tomatoes, halved
- 1/2 cup fresh basil leaves, chopped
- 1/4 cup crumbled feta cheese
- 2 tablespoons extra virgin olive oil
- 2 tablespoons balsamic vinegar
- 1 teaspoon Dijon mustard
- 1 clove garlic, minced
- Salt and pepper to taste

1. Cook the farro according to package instructions. Drain and let cool slightly.

2. In a large bowl, combine the cooked farro, halved tomatoes, chopped basil, and crumbled feta.

3. In a small bowl, whisk together the olive oil, balsamic vinegar, Dijon mustard, and minced garlic. Season with salt and pepper.

4. Pour the dressing over the farro salad and toss gently to coat.

5. Let the salad sit for 10-15 minutes to allow the flavors to meld.

6. Serve the farro salad at room temperature or chilled.

This farro salad is an excellent choice for a menopause-friendly diet. Farro is a whole grain that is high in fiber, protein, and minerals. Tomatoes provide lycopene, which may help reduce hot flashes. The fresh basil and balsamic vinegar dressing add flavor and antioxidants.

The crumbled feta cheese provides calcium, which is important for bone health during menopause. This salad can be enjoyed as a main dish or a side. It's a nutritious and delicious way to incorporate more plant-based foods into your diet.

How would you rate this dish?

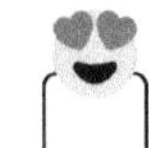 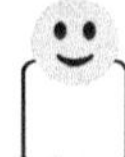 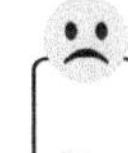 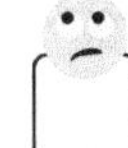 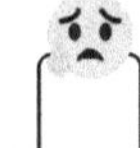

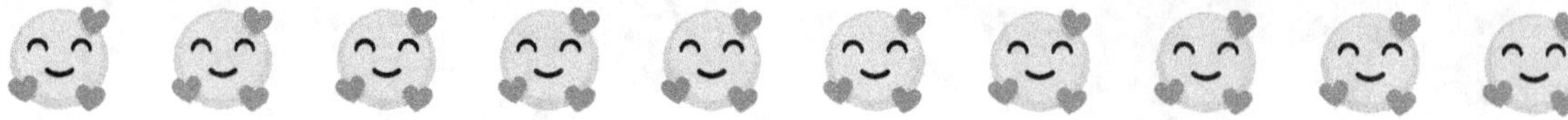

77. Watermelon and Feta Salad

 Prep Time : 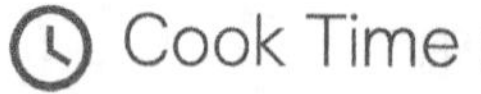 Cook Time : 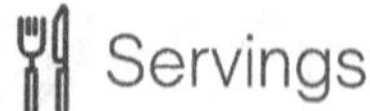 Servings :

Is this dish easy or difficult for you to make?

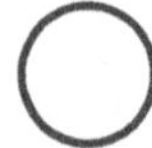 ◯ 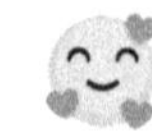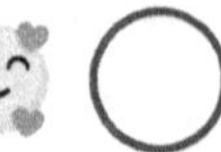 ◯

Write 5 friends with whom you want to share this dish

....

....

....

....

....

INGREDIENTS

- 4 cups cubed seedless watermelon
- 1 cup crumbled feta cheese
- 1/4 cup thinly sliced red onion
- 1/4 cup chopped fresh mint
- 2 tablespoons balsamic glaze
- 1 tablespoon extra virgin olive oil
- Juice of 1 lime
- Salt and pepper to taste

1. In a large bowl, gently combine the cubed watermelon, crumbled feta cheese, sliced red onion, and chopped fresh mint.

2. Drizzle the balsamic glaze and olive oil over the salad. Squeeze the lime juice on top.

3. Gently toss the salad to coat the ingredients evenly.

4. Season with salt and pepper to taste.

5. Serve the watermelon and feta salad immediately or chill in the refrigerator for 30 minutes before serving.

This refreshing watermelon salad is an excellent choice for a menopause-friendly diet. Watermelon is high in water content, which can help with hydration, and it also contains lycopene, an antioxidant that may help reduce hot flashes.

The feta cheese provides calcium, which is important for bone health during menopause. The red onion and mint add flavor and anti-inflammatory properties.

The balsamic glaze and lime juice dressing complement the sweetness of the watermelon and provide a tangy, flavorful contrast.

This salad is a great option for a light and healthy summer meal or side dish. Enjoy the combination of sweet, salty, and refreshing flavors!

How would you rate this dish?

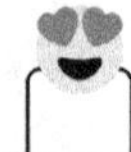 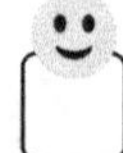 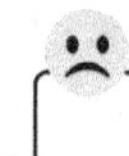 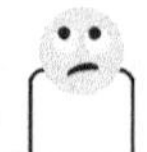 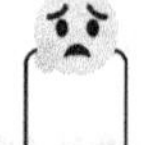

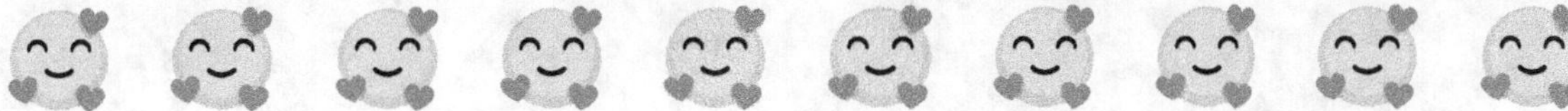

78. Caprese Salad with Mozzarella and Basil

 Prep Time :    Cook Time :   Servings :

Is this dish easy or difficult for you to make?

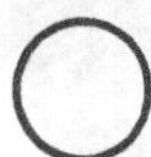 ◯   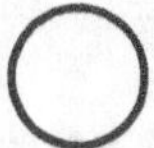 ◯

Write 5 friends with whom you want to share this dish

INGREDIENTS

- 8 oz fresh mozzarella cheese, sliced
- 3 medium tomatoes, sliced
- 1/4 cup fresh basil leaves
- 2 tablespoons extra virgin olive oil
- 1 tablespoon balsamic vinegar
- Salt and freshly ground black pepper to taste

1. Arrange the sliced mozzarella and tomatoes on a serving platter or plate in an overlapping pattern.

2. Scatter the fresh basil leaves over the top.

3. Drizzle the olive oil and balsamic vinegar evenly over the salad.

4. Season generously with salt and freshly ground black pepper.

5. Let the salad sit for 5-10 minutes to allow the flavors to meld.

6. Serve immediately.

Tips:
- Use the freshest, ripest tomatoes you can find for the best flavor.
- For extra creaminess, you can add a dollop of high-quality balsamic glaze over the top.
- Garnish with a sprinkle of flaky sea salt if desired.
- This salad pairs beautifully with crusty bread or grilled chicken or fish.

The classic combination of juicy tomatoes, creamy mozzarella, and fragrant basil makes this Caprese salad a simple yet delicious summer dish. Enjoy!

How would you rate this dish?

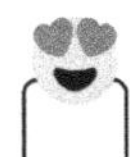  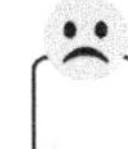 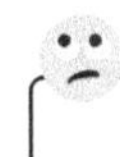 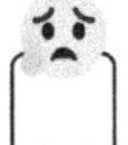

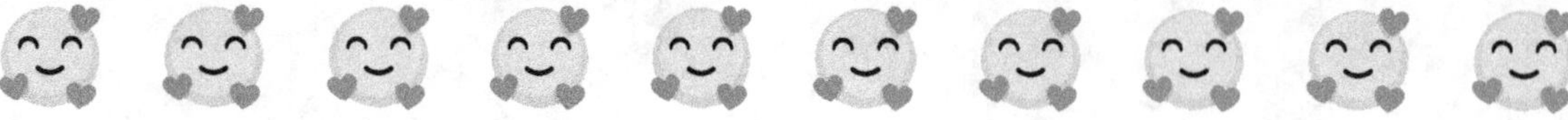

79. Tuna Salad with Avocado and Cucumbers

Let's do that and fill in the time here

 Prep Time : 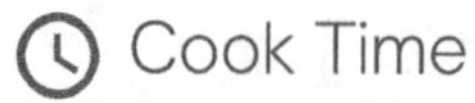 Cook Time :  Servings :

Write 5 friends with whom you want to share this dish

....

....

....

....

....

Is this dish easy or difficult for you to make?

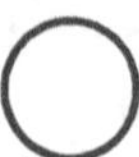 ◯   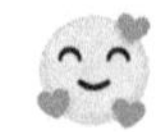 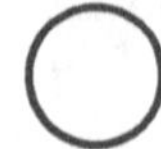 ◯

INGREDIENTS

- 2 (5 oz) cans of tuna, drained
- 1 avocado, diced
- 1 cucumber, diced
- 2 tablespoons plain Greek yogurt
- 1 tablespoon lemon juice
- 1 tablespoon chopped fresh dill (or 1 tsp dried dill)
- Salt and pepper to taste
- Lettuce leaves or whole grain crackers, for serving

1. In a medium bowl, gently mix together the drained tuna, diced avocado, and diced cucumber.

2. Add the Greek yogurt, lemon juice, and chopped fresh dill (or dried dill). Stir to combine.

3. Season the tuna salad with salt and pepper to taste.

4. Serve the tuna salad on a bed of lettuce leaves or with whole grain crackers.

This tuna salad is a great option for a healthy and satisfying meal or snack. The combination of tuna, avocado, and cucumber provides a nice balance of protein, healthy fats, and fresh crunch.

The Greek yogurt adds creaminess and a boost of protein, while the lemon juice and dill provide bright, refreshing flavors. This tuna salad is perfect for enjoying on its own or using as a topping for greens, sandwiches, or crackers.

This recipe is a great choice for a menopause-friendly diet, as it is packed with nutrients that can help support overall health during this transition, such as omega-3 fatty acids, antioxidants, and fiber.

Enjoy this delicious and nutritious tuna salad!

How would you rate this dish?

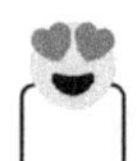 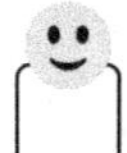 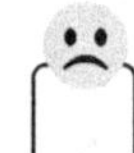 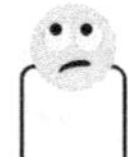 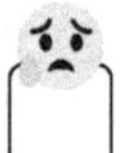

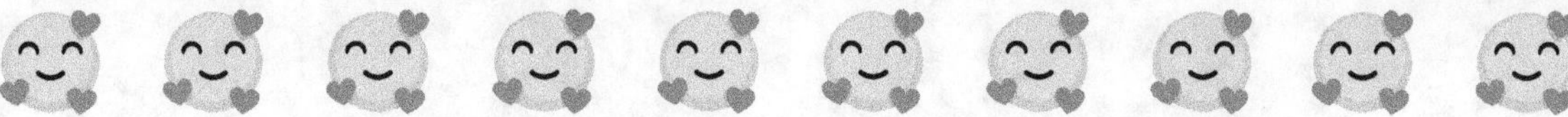

80. Roasted Beet and Arugula Salad

 Prep Time :   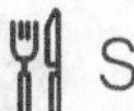 Cook Time :   Servings :

Let's do that and fill in the time here

Is this dish easy or difficult for you to make?

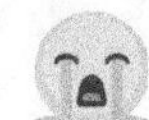 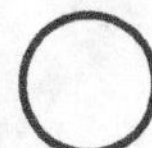 ◯   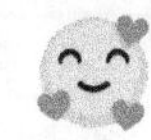 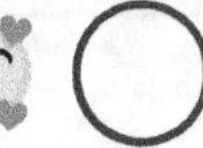 ◯

Write 5 friends with whom you want to share this dish

....

....

....

....

....

INGREDIENTS

- 3 medium beets, peeled and cut into 1-inch cubes
- 2 tablespoons olive oil
- Salt and pepper to taste
- 5 oz baby arugula
- 1/4 cup crumbled feta cheese
- 2 tablespoons toasted walnuts
- 2 tablespoons balsamic vinegar
- 1 tablespoon Dijon mustard
- 1 teaspoon honey

1. Preheat your oven to 400°F.

2. Toss the cubed beets with the olive oil and season with salt and pepper.

3. Spread the beets in a single layer on a baking sheet. Roast for 25-30 minutes, stirring halfway, until the beets are tender and lightly caramelized.

4. Allow the roasted beets to cool slightly.

5. In a large salad bowl, combine the baby arugula, roasted beets, crumbled feta cheese, and toasted walnuts.

6. In a small bowl, whisk together the balsamic vinegar, Dijon mustard, and honey to make the dressing.

7. Drizzle the balsamic dressing over the salad and toss gently to coat.

8. Serve the roasted beet and arugula salad immediately.

This salad is a delicious and nutritious option. The roasted beets provide a sweet, earthy flavor and are packed with vitamins and minerals. The peppery arugula, creamy feta, and crunchy walnuts create a wonderful contrast of textures and flavors.

The balsamic vinaigrette ties everything together with its tangy and slightly sweet notes. This salad is a great choice for a menopause-friendly diet, as it is rich in antioxidants, fiber, and healthy fats.

How would you rate this dish?

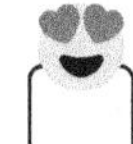 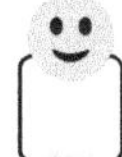  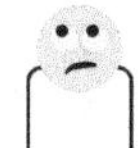 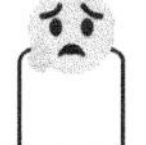

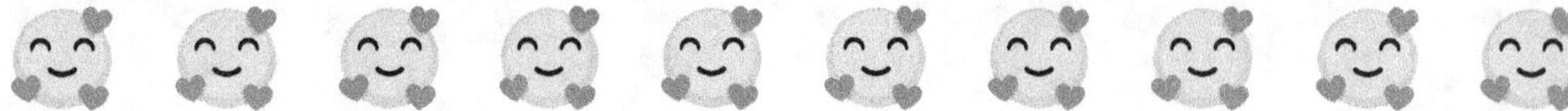

81. Grilled Chicken Breast with Quinoa and Green Beans

 Prep Time :   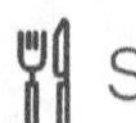 Cook Time :   Servings :

Write 5 friends with whom you want to share this dish

....

....

....

....

....

Is this dish easy or difficult for you to make?

 ◯   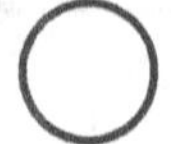 ◯

INGREDIENTS

- 4 boneless, skinless chicken breasts
- 1 cup uncooked quinoa, rinsed
- 2 cups low-sodium chicken or vegetable broth
- 1 lb fresh green beans, trimmed
- 2 tablespoons olive oil, divided
- 1 teaspoon dried thyme
- 1 teaspoon garlic powder
- Salt and pepper to taste
- Lemon wedges for serving

1. Preheat grill or grill pan to medium-high heat.

2. In a medium saucepan, combine the quinoa and broth. Bring to a boil, then reduce heat to low, cover, and simmer for 15-20 minutes until quinoa is tender. Fluff with a fork.

3. In a large skillet, heat 1 tablespoon of olive oil over medium-high heat. Add the green beans and sauté for 5-7 minutes until tender-crisp. Season with salt and pepper.

4. Brush the chicken breasts with the remaining 1 tablespoon of olive oil and season with the thyme, garlic powder, salt, and pepper.

5. Grill the chicken for 5-7 minutes per side, or until cooked through and no longer pink in the center.

6. Serve the grilled chicken breast over the cooked quinoa, accompanied by the sautéed green beans. Garnish with lemon wedges.

This grilled chicken, quinoa, and green bean dish is an excellent choice for a menopause-friendly diet. Chicken is a lean protein that provides essential amino acids. Quinoa is a whole grain that is high in fiber, protein, and minerals. Green beans are a nutrient-dense vegetable that can help support overall health during menopause.

The combination of lean protein, complex carbohydrates, and fiber-rich vegetables makes this a balanced and satisfying meal. Enjoy!

How would you rate this dish?

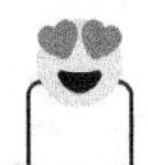 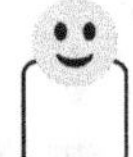 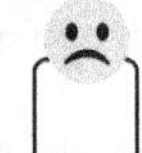 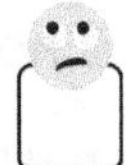 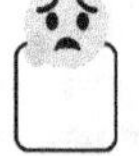 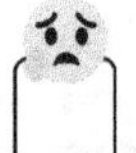

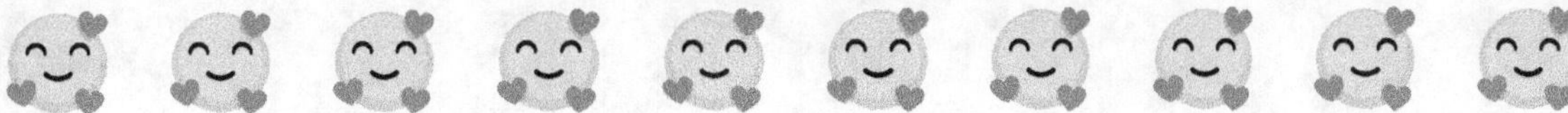

82. Baked Salmon with Lemon and Dill

 Prep Time :

 Cook Time :

Servings :

Write 5 friends with whom you want to share this dish

INGREDIENTS

- 4 (6 oz) salmon fillets
- 2 tablespoons olive oil
- 2 tablespoons freshly squeezed lemon juice
- 2 teaspoons dried dill
- 1 teaspoon grated lemon zest
- Salt and pepper to taste
- Lemon wedges for serving

Is this dish easy or difficult for you to make?

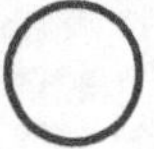 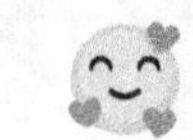 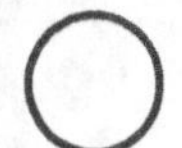

1. Preheat your oven to 400°F. Line a baking sheet with parchment paper or foil.

2. Place the salmon fillets on the prepared baking sheet.

3. In a small bowl, whisk together the olive oil, lemon juice, dried dill, and lemon zest.

4. Brush the salmon fillets evenly with the lemon-dill mixture, making sure to coat the tops and sides.

5. Season the salmon with salt and pepper.

6. Bake the salmon for 12-15 minutes, or until it flakes easily with a fork and is cooked through.

7. Serve the baked salmon warm, with lemon wedges on the side.

This baked salmon dish is an excellent choice for a menopause-friendly diet. Salmon is a rich source of omega-3 fatty acids, which can help reduce inflammation and may alleviate some menopausal symptoms.

The lemon and dill provide bright, fresh flavors that complement the salmon without the need for heavy sauces or seasonings. Lemon is also a good source of vitamin C, which can help support the immune system during menopause.

This simple, yet delicious, salmon recipe is easy to prepare and pairs well with a variety of side dishes, such as roasted vegetables or a fresh salad. Enjoy this nutritious and flavorful meal!

How would you rate this dish?

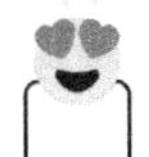  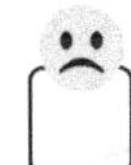 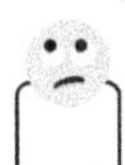 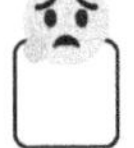

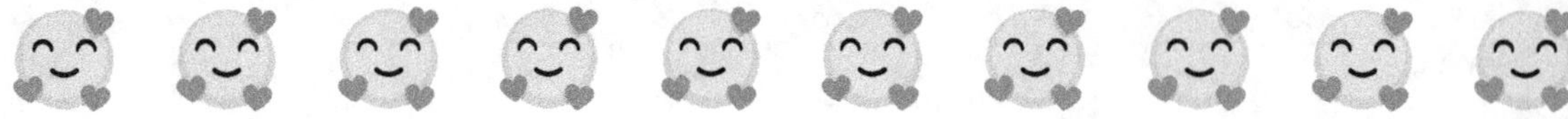

83. Stuffed Peppers with Ground Turkey and Brown Rice

Let's do that and fill in the time here

 Prep Time : 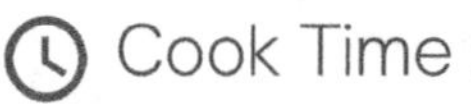

 Cook Time :

Servings :

Write 5 friends with whom you want to share this dish

....

....

....

....

....

Is this dish easy or difficult for you to make?

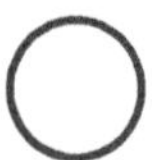 ◯　　　 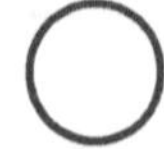 ◯

INGREDIENTS

- 6 bell peppers (any color)
- 1 lb ground turkey
- 1 cup cooked brown rice
- 1 small onion, diced
- 3 cloves garlic, minced
- 1 (14.5 oz) can diced tomatoes
- 1 teaspoon dried oregano
- 1 teaspoon dried basil
- 1/2 teaspoon red pepper flakes (optional)
- Salt and pepper to taste
- 1 cup shredded mozzarella cheese

1. Preheat your oven to 375°F.

2. Cut the tops off the bell peppers and remove the seeds and membranes. Place the peppers in a baking dish.

3. In a large skillet, cook the ground turkey over medium heat, breaking it up as it cooks, until no longer pink, about 5-7 minutes. Drain any excess fat.

4. Add the onion and garlic to the skillet and cook for 2-3 minutes until fragrant.

5. Stir in the cooked brown rice, diced tomatoes, oregano, basil, red pepper flakes (if using), and season with salt and pepper.

6. Spoon the turkey and rice mixture into the hollowed-out bell peppers, packing it in tightly.

7. Top each stuffed pepper with shredded mozzarella cheese.

8. Cover the baking dish with foil and bake for 30-35 minutes, until the peppers are tender.

9. Remove the foil and bake for an additional 5-10 minutes, until the cheese is melted and lightly browned. Serve the stuffed peppers warm.

These stuffed peppers are a delicious and nutritious meal. The ground turkey provides lean protein, while the brown rice and bell peppers offer complex carbohydrates, fiber, and a variety of vitamins and minerals. This dish is a great option for a balanced, menopause-friendly diet.

How would you rate this dish?

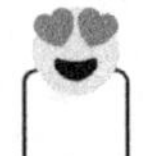 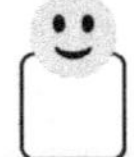 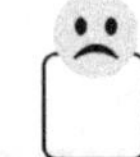 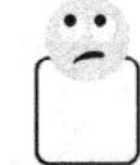 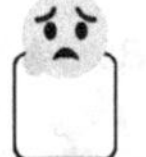

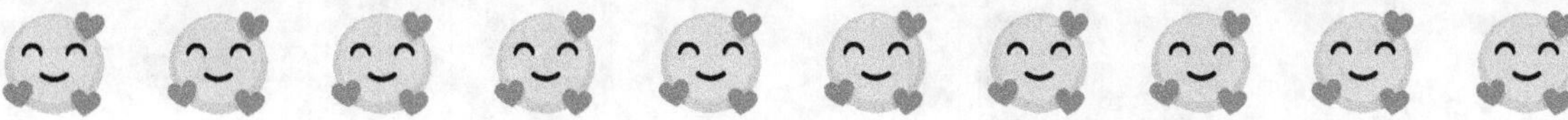

84. Vegetable Stir-Fry with Tofu

Let's do that and fill in the time here

Prep Time :

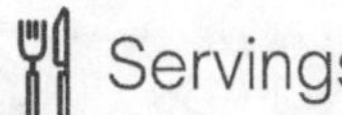
Cook Time :

Servings :

Is this dish easy or difficult for you to make?

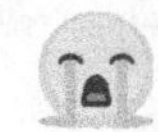 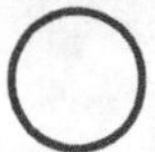 ⚪   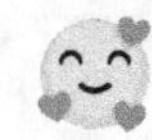  ⚪

Write 5 friends with whom you want to share this dish

....

....

....

....

....

INGREDIENTS

- 1 block (14 oz) extra-firm tofu, cubed
- 2 tablespoons sesame oil, divided
- 2 cups broccoli florets
- 1 red bell pepper, sliced
- 1 cup sliced mushrooms
- 1 cup snow peas or snap peas
- 3 cloves garlic, minced
- 1 tablespoon grated fresh ginger
- 2 tablespoons low-sodium soy sauce or tamari
- 1 tablespoon rice vinegar
- 1 teaspoon sesame seeds (optional)
- Salt and pepper to taste
- Cooked brown rice, for serving

1. In a large skillet or wok, heat 1 tablespoon of sesame oil over medium-high heat. Add the cubed tofu and sauté for 5-7 minutes, turning occasionally, until lightly browned on all sides. Transfer the tofu to a plate and set aside.

2. In the same skillet, heat the remaining 1 tablespoon of sesame oil. Add the broccoli, bell pepper, mushrooms, and snow peas. Sauté for 5-7 minutes, stirring frequently, until the vegetables are tender-crisp.

3. Add the garlic and ginger to the skillet and cook for 1 minute, until fragrant.

4. Return the sautéed tofu to the skillet. Pour in the soy sauce and rice vinegar. Toss everything together until well combined and heated through.

5. Remove from heat and sprinkle with sesame seeds, if using. Season with salt and pepper to taste. Serve the vegetable stir-fry over cooked brown rice.

This vegetable stir-fry with tofu is an excellent choice for a menopause-friendly diet. Tofu is a plant-based protein that is rich in isoflavones, which can help alleviate some menopausal symptoms. The variety of vegetables provides a range of vitamins, minerals, and antioxidants that support overall health during this transition.

The ginger and soy sauce add flavor and anti-inflammatory properties to the dish. Serve this stir-fry with a side of nutrient-dense brown rice for a complete and satisfying meal.

How would you rate this dish?

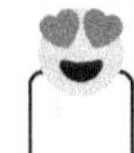 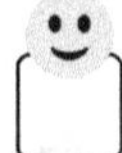 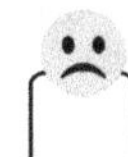 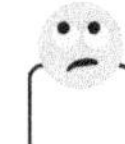 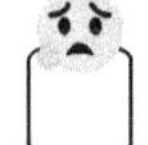

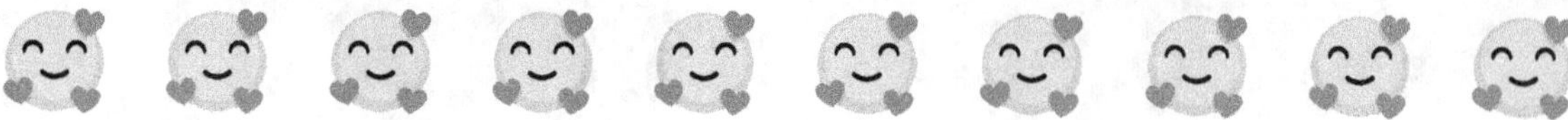

85. Baked Cod with Garlic and Herbs

 Prep Time :    Cook Time :   Servings :

Is this dish easy or difficult for you to make?

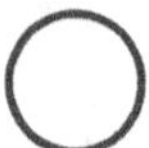 ◯   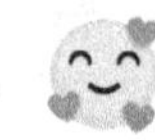 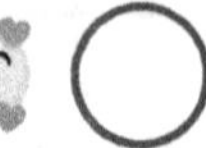 ◯

Write 5 friends with whom you want to share this dish ....

INGREDIENTS

- 4 (6 oz) cod fillets
- 2 tablespoons olive oil
- 3 cloves garlic, minced
- 2 tablespoons chopped fresh parsley
- 1 tablespoon chopped fresh dill
- 1 teaspoon grated lemon zest
- Salt and pepper to taste
- Lemon wedges for serving

1. Preheat your oven to 400°F. Lightly grease a baking dish or line it with parchment paper.

2. Place the cod fillets in the prepared baking dish.

3. In a small bowl, combine the olive oil, minced garlic, chopped parsley, chopped dill, and lemon zest. Mix well.

4. Spoon the garlic-herb mixture evenly over the top of the cod fillets, making sure to coat them completely.

5. Season the cod with salt and pepper.

6. Bake the cod for 12-15 minutes, or until it flakes easily with a fork and is opaque throughout.

7. Serve the baked cod immediately, with lemon wedges on the side.

This baked cod dish is an excellent choice for a menopause-friendly diet. Cod is a lean, flaky white fish that is high in protein and low in mercury, making it a safe choice for women during this transition.

The garlic, herbs, and lemon provide a flavorful and aromatic topping that complements the cod without the need for heavy sauces or seasonings. Garlic and herbs are also known for their anti-inflammatory properties, which can be beneficial during menopause.

How would you rate this dish?

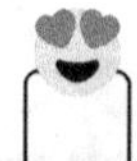 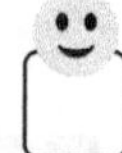  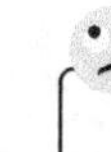 

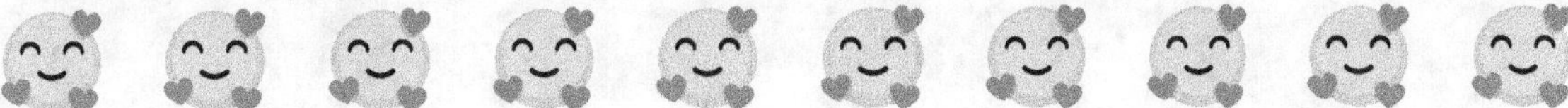

86. Chicken Fajitas with Bell Peppers and Onions

 *Let's do that and fill in the time here* 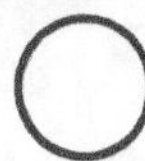 Prep Time :  Cook Time : 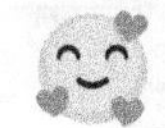 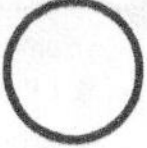 Servings :

Write 5 friends with whom you want to share this dish

....

....

....

....

....

Is this dish easy or difficult for you to make?

😭 ◯   🙂 ◯

INGREDIENTS

- 1 lb boneless, skinless chicken breasts, sliced into strips
- 2 bell peppers (any color), sliced into strips
- 1 onion, sliced into strips
- 2 tablespoons olive oil
- 2 teaspoons chili powder
- 1 teaspoon cumin
- 1 teaspoon garlic powder
- Salt and pepper to taste
- 8-10 small whole wheat tortillas or lettuce wraps
- Toppings: avocado, salsa, plain Greek yogurt, chopped cilantro

1. In a large skillet or wok, heat the olive oil over medium-high heat.

2. Add the sliced chicken, bell peppers, and onions. Season with the chili powder, cumin, garlic powder, salt, and pepper.

3. Sauté the mixture, stirring occasionally, for 8-10 minutes until the chicken is cooked through and the vegetables are tender-crisp.

4. Warm the tortillas or prepare the lettuce wraps.

5. Serve the chicken fajita filling in the tortillas or lettuce wraps, allowing everyone to customize their own with the desired toppings.

This chicken fajita recipe is an excellent choice for a menopause-friendly diet. Chicken is a lean protein that provides essential amino acids. Bell peppers are rich in vitamin C, which can help reduce hot flashes, while onions contain anti-inflammatory compounds.

The whole wheat tortillas or lettuce wraps provide complex carbohydrates and fiber, which can help regulate blood sugar levels. Avocado, salsa, and Greek yogurt add healthy fats, vitamins, and probiotics to support overall health during menopause.

This dish is easy to prepare, full of flavor, and provides a balanced, nutrient-dense meal. Enjoy!

How would you rate this dish?

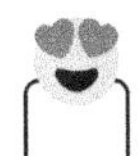 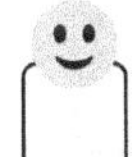 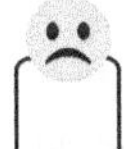 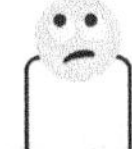 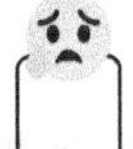

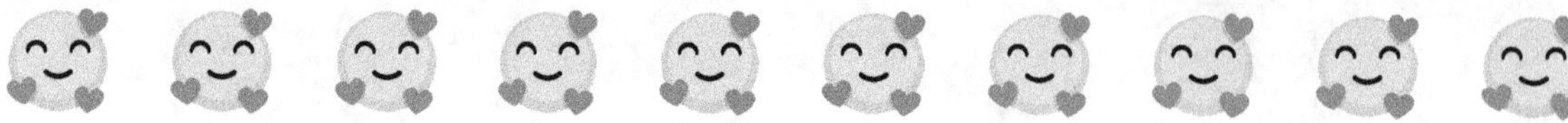

87. Shrimp Tacos with Avocado and Cilantro

 Prep Time :

Cook Time :

Servings :

Write 5 friends with whom you want to share this dish

....

....

....

....

....

Is this dish easy or difficult for you to make?

 ◯   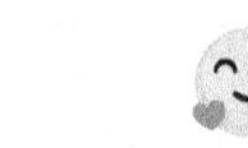 ◯ 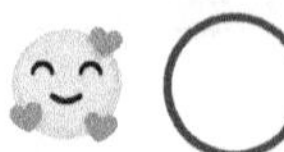 ◯

INGREDIENTS

- 1 lb shrimp, peeled and deveined
- 2 tablespoons olive oil
- 1 teaspoon chili powder
- 1/2 teaspoon cumin
- Salt and pepper to taste
- 8-10 small whole wheat tortillas
- 1 avocado, diced
- 1/4 cup chopped fresh cilantro
- 1 lime, cut into wedges
- Optional toppings: shredded cabbage, diced tomatoes, plain Greek yogurt

1. In a large skillet, heat the olive oil over medium-high heat.

2. Add the shrimp to the skillet and season with the chili powder, cumin, salt, and pepper. Sauté the shrimp for 3-5 minutes, until they are opaque and cooked through.

3. Remove the skillet from heat and transfer the cooked shrimp to a plate.

4. Warm the whole wheat tortillas according to package instructions.

5. To assemble the tacos, place a few pieces of shrimp in each tortilla. Top with diced avocado and chopped fresh cilantro.

6. Serve the shrimp tacos with lime wedges on the side. Additional toppings like shredded cabbage, diced tomatoes, and a dollop of plain Greek yogurt can be added if desired.

These shrimp tacos are an excellent choice for a menopause-friendly diet. Shrimp is a lean protein that provides essential amino acids, while the avocado offers healthy fats and fiber. The cilantro and lime add fresh, vibrant flavors and antioxidants.

The whole wheat tortillas provide complex carbohydrates and fiber, which can help regulate blood sugar levels. The optional toppings, such as cabbage and Greek yogurt, further enhance the nutritional profile of this dish

How would you rate this dish?

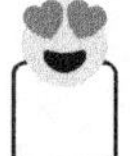 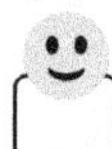 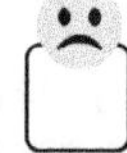 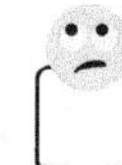 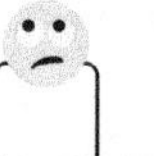 

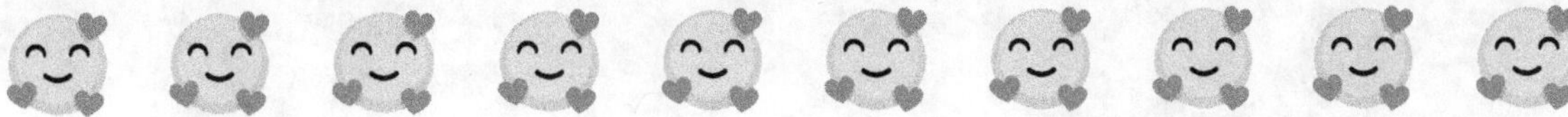

88. Grilled Portobello Mushrooms with Balsamic Glaze

 Prep Time :

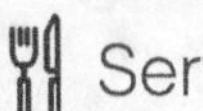 Cook Time :

Servings :

Is this dish easy or difficult for you to make?

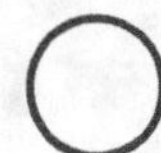 ◯ 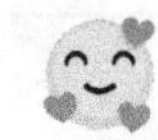 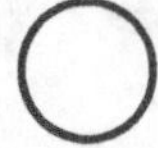 ◯

Write 5 friends with whom you want to share this dish

....

....

....

....

....

INGREDIENTS

- 4 large portobello mushroom caps, stems removed
- 2 tablespoons olive oil
- 2 tablespoons balsamic vinegar
- 1 tablespoon honey
- 2 cloves garlic, minced
- 1 teaspoon dried thyme
- Salt and pepper to taste
- Chopped fresh parsley for garnish (optional)

1. Preheat your grill or grill pan to medium-high heat.

2. In a small bowl, whisk together the olive oil, balsamic vinegar, honey, minced garlic, and dried thyme. Season with salt and pepper.

3. Brush the portobello mushroom caps on both sides with the balsamic glaze mixture, reserving any remaining glaze.

4. Grill the mushrooms for 4-5 minutes per side, or until they are tender and lightly charred.

5. Transfer the grilled portobello mushrooms to a serving plate.

6. Drizzle the remaining balsamic glaze over the top of the mushrooms.

7. Garnish with chopped fresh parsley, if desired.

8. Serve the grilled portobello mushrooms warm.

These grilled portobello mushrooms are an excellent choice for a menopause-friendly diet. Portobello mushrooms are a good source of antioxidants, such as selenium and vitamin D, which can help support overall health during menopause.

The balsamic glaze provides a tangy and slightly sweet flavor, while the garlic and thyme add depth and anti-inflammatory properties to the dish.

This simple, yet flavorful, recipe can be enjoyed as a main course or a side dish. Pair it with a fresh salad or roasted vegetables for a complete and nutritious meal.

How would you rate this dish?

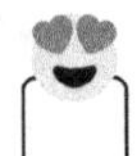 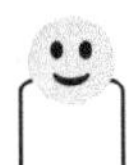 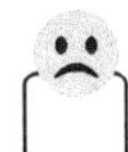 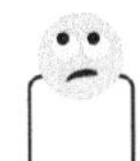 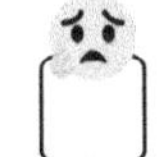

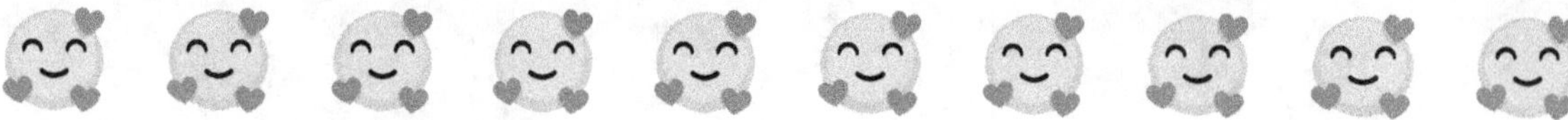

89. Turkey Meatballs with Marinara Sauce

 *Let's do that and fill in the time here* (✓) Prep Time : 〇 Cook Time : 🍴 Servings : 

Is this dish easy or difficult for you to make?

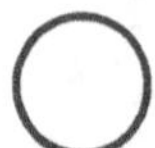 〇  〇

Write 5 friends with whom you want to share this dish

....

....

....

....

....

INGREDIENTS

- 1 lb ground turkey
- 1/2 cup whole wheat breadcrumbs
- 1/4 cup grated Parmesan cheese
- 1 egg, lightly beaten
- 2 cloves garlic, minced
- 2 tablespoons chopped fresh parsley
- 1 teaspoon dried oregano
- 1/2 teaspoon salt
- 1/4 teaspoon black pepper
- 1 (24 oz) jar low-sodium marinara sauce
- Cooked whole wheat pasta, for serving

1. Preheat your oven to 400°F. Line a baking sheet with parchment paper.

2. In a large bowl, combine the ground turkey, breadcrumbs, Parmesan cheese, egg, garlic, parsley, oregano, salt, and pepper. Mix until well incorporated.

3. Roll the mixture into 1-inch meatballs and place them on the prepared baking sheet.

4. Bake the meatballs for 18-20 minutes, or until they are cooked through and no longer pink in the center.

5. In a saucepan, heat the marinara sauce over medium heat until simmering.

6. Add the baked meatballs to the marinara sauce and gently stir to coat.

7. Serve the turkey meatballs and marinara sauce over cooked whole wheat pasta.

This turkey meatball dish is an excellent choice for a menopause-friendly diet. Ground turkey is a lean protein that provides essential amino acids. The whole wheat breadcrumbs and pasta offer complex carbohydrates and fiber, which can help regulate blood sugar levels.

The Parmesan cheese adds a boost of calcium, while the herbs and spices provide anti-inflammatory benefits. The low-sodium marinara sauce is a good source of lycopene, an antioxidant that may help reduce hot flashes.

How would you rate this dish?

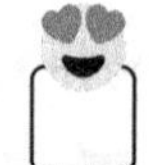 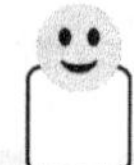 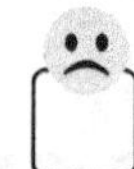 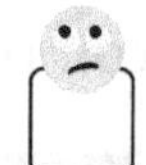 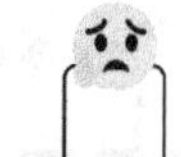

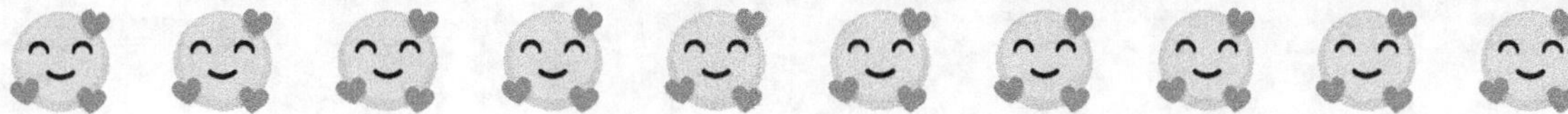

90. Vegetable Paella with Brown Rice

 Prep Time :  Cook Time : Servings :

Is this dish easy or difficult for you to make?

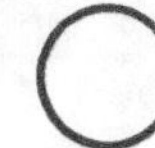 ◯ 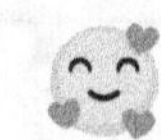 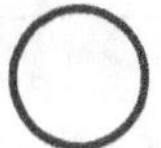 ◯

Write 5 friends with whom you want to share this dish

....

....

....

....

....

INGREDIENTS

- 1 cup uncooked brown rice
- 2 cups low-sodium vegetable broth
- 1 tablespoon olive oil
- 1 onion, diced
- 3 cloves garlic, minced
- 1 red bell pepper, diced
- 1 cup sliced mushrooms
- 1 cup frozen peas
- 1 teaspoon smoked paprika
- 1/2 teaspoon saffron threads (optional)
- 1/4 teaspoon cayenne pepper (optional)
- Salt and pepper to taste
- Chopped parsley for garnish

1. In a medium saucepan, combine the brown rice and vegetable broth. Bring to a boil, then reduce heat, cover, and simmer for 25-30 minutes, until the rice is tender. Fluff with a fork.

2. In a large skillet or paella pan, heat the olive oil over medium heat. Add the diced onion and sauté for 5 minutes until translucent.

3. Add the minced garlic, diced bell pepper, sliced mushrooms, and frozen peas. Cook for 5-7 minutes, stirring occasionally, until the vegetables are tender.

4. Stir in the cooked brown rice, smoked paprika, saffron (if using), and cayenne (if using). Season with salt and pepper.

5. Cook for an additional 5 minutes, stirring occasionally, to allow the flavors to meld.

6. Remove from heat and garnish the vegetable paella with chopped parsley.

7. Serve the paella warm.

This vegetable paella is an excellent choice for a menopause-friendly diet. Brown rice provides complex carbohydrates and fiber, which can help regulate blood sugar levels. The variety of vegetables, such as bell peppers, mushrooms, and peas, offer a range of vitamins, minerals, and antioxidants that support overall health during menopause.

How would you rate this dish?

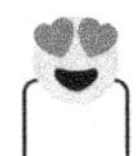  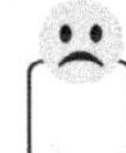 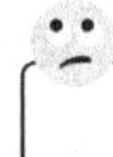 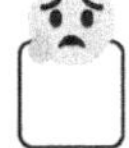

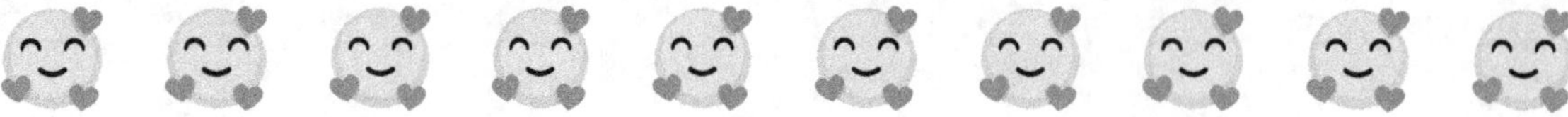

91. Roasted Brussels Sprouts with Balsamic Glaze

 Prep Time : 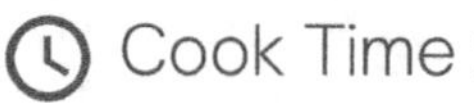  Cook Time : Servings :

Is this dish easy or difficult for you to make?

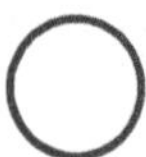 ◯   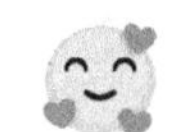 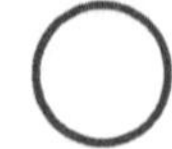 ◯

Write 5 friends with whom you want to share this dish

....

....

....

....

....

INGREDIENTS

- 1 lb Brussels sprouts, trimmed and halved
- 2 tablespoons olive oil
- 1/4 cup balsamic vinegar
- 2 tablespoons honey
- 1 teaspoon Dijon mustard
- Salt and pepper to taste
- Chopped fresh parsley for garnish (optional)

1. Preheat your oven to 400°F. Line a baking sheet with parchment paper.

2. In a large bowl, toss the trimmed and halved Brussels sprouts with the olive oil. Season with salt and pepper.

3. Spread the Brussels sprouts in a single layer on the prepared baking sheet.

4. Roast the Brussels sprouts for 20-25 minutes, tossing halfway, until they are tender and lightly browned.

5. In a small saucepan, combine the balsamic vinegar and honey. Bring the mixture to a simmer over medium heat, stirring occasionally, until it thickens slightly, about 5 minutes.

6. Remove the balsamic glaze from heat and stir in the Dijon mustard.

7. Transfer the roasted Brussels sprouts to a serving bowl. Drizzle the balsamic glaze over the top and toss gently to coat.

8. Garnish the Brussels sprouts with chopped fresh parsley, if desired.

9. Serve the roasted Brussels sprouts with balsamic glaze warm.

The balsamic glaze provides a tangy and slightly sweet flavor, while the Dijon mustard adds a touch of creaminess. This combination of flavors complements the nutty, caramelized Brussels sprouts

How would you rate this dish?

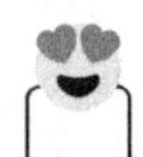 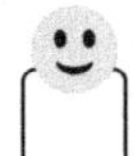 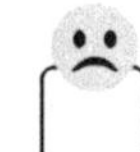 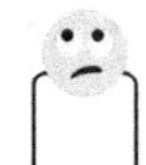 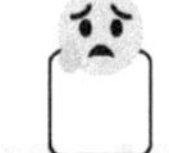

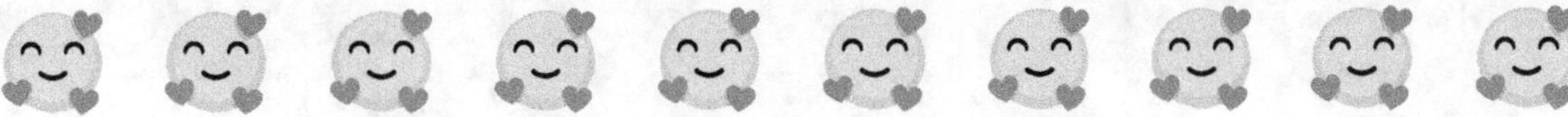

92. Garlic Mashed Cauliflower

 Prep Time :   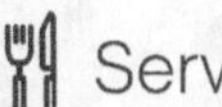 Cook Time :   Servings :

Is this dish easy or difficult for you to make?

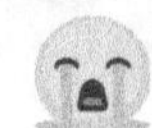 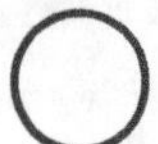 ◯   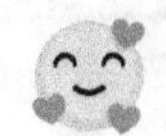  ◯

Write 5 friends with whom you want to share this dish

INGREDIENTS

- 1 large head of cauliflower, cut into florets
- 2 tablespoons unsweetened almond milk
- 2 tablespoons olive oil
- 3 cloves garlic, minced
- 1/4 cup grated Parmesan cheese (optional)
- Salt and pepper to taste
- Chopped fresh parsley for garnish (optional)

1. In a large pot, bring a few inches of water to a boil. Add the cauliflower florets and steam for 10-12 minutes, until very tender.

2. Drain the cauliflower and transfer it to a food processor or high-powered blender.

3. Add the almond milk, olive oil, and minced garlic to the food processor. Blend until the mixture is smooth and creamy, scraping down the sides as needed.

4. If using, stir in the grated Parmesan cheese until well combined.

5. Season the mashed cauliflower with salt and pepper to taste.

6. Transfer the garlic mashed cauliflower to a serving bowl and garnish with chopped fresh parsley, if desired.

7. Serve the mashed cauliflower warm.

This garlic mashed cauliflower is an excellent choice for a menopause-friendly diet. Cauliflower is a cruciferous vegetable that is high in fiber, vitamins, and antioxidants, which can help support overall health during menopause.

The garlic provides anti-inflammatory benefits, while the optional Parmesan cheese adds a creamy texture and a boost of calcium. The almond milk makes this dish dairy-free, which can be beneficial for some women during this transition.

How would you rate this dish?

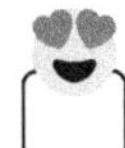 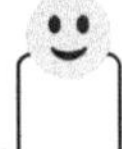 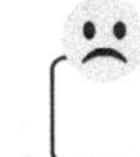 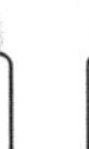 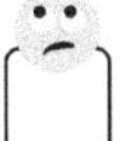 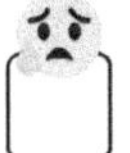

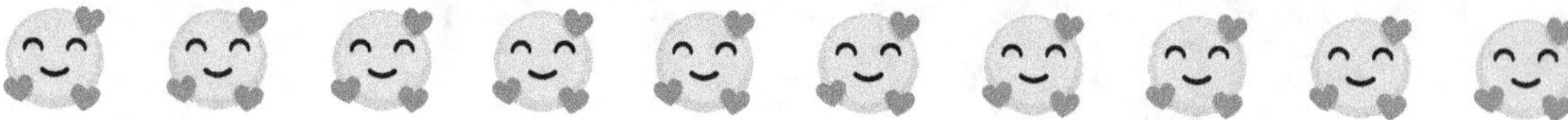

93. Quinoa with Dried Cranberries and Pecans

Let's do that and fill in the time here

 Prep Time :   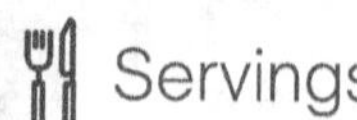 Cook Time :   Servings :

Write 5 friends with whom you want to share this dish
....
....
....
....
....

INGREDIENTS

- 1 cup uncooked quinoa, rinsed
- 2 cups low-sodium vegetable or chicken broth
- 1/2 cup dried cranberries
- 1/4 cup chopped pecans
- 2 tablespoons chopped fresh parsley
- 1 tablespoon olive oil
- 1 tablespoon balsamic vinegar
- 1/4 teaspoon ground cinnamon
- Salt and pepper to taste

Is this dish easy or difficult for you to make?

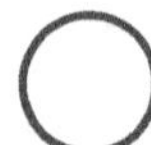 ◯   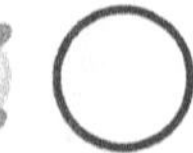 ◯

1. In a medium saucepan, combine the rinsed quinoa and broth. Bring to a boil, then reduce heat, cover, and simmer for 15-20 minutes, until the quinoa is tender and the liquid is absorbed.

2. Remove the quinoa from heat and fluff with a fork. Allow it to cool slightly.

3. In a large bowl, combine the cooked quinoa, dried cranberries, chopped pecans, and chopped fresh parsley.

4. In a small bowl, whisk together the olive oil, balsamic vinegar, and ground cinnamon.

5. Drizzle the dressing over the quinoa mixture and toss gently to coat.

6. Season the quinoa salad with salt and pepper to taste.

7. Serve the quinoa with dried cranberries and pecans at room temperature or chilled.

This quinoa dish is a great option for a menopause-friendly diet. Quinoa is a whole grain that is high in protein, fiber, and minerals. The dried cranberries provide a sweet-tart flavor and antioxidants, while the pecans add healthy fats and crunch.

The balsamic vinaigrette dressing complements the other ingredients nicely, and the cinnamon adds a warm, comforting note.

How would you rate this dish?

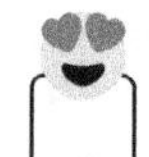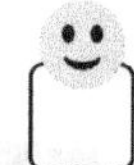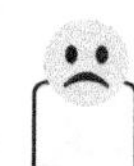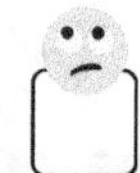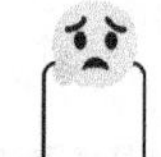

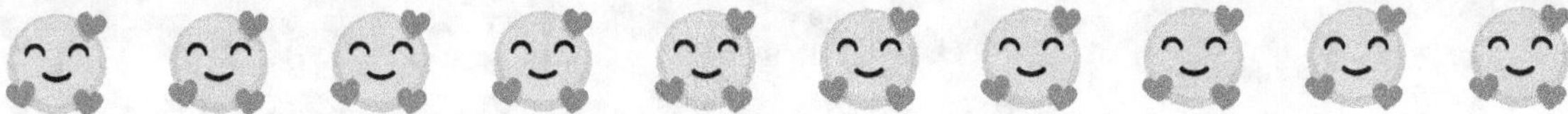

94. Steamed Asparagus with Lemon Zest

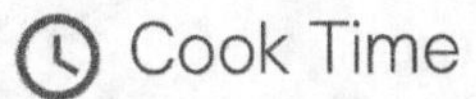 Prep Time :　　Cook Time :　　Servings :

Is this dish easy or difficult for you to make?

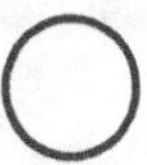 ◯　　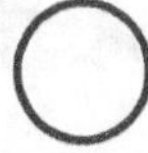 ◯

Write 5 friends with whom you want to share this dish

....

....

....

....

....

INGREDIENTS

- 1 lb fresh asparagus, trimmed
- 1 tablespoon olive oil
- 1 tablespoon lemon zest
- 1 tablespoon lemon juice
- Salt and pepper to taste

1. Fill a large pot with about 1 inch of water and bring it to a boil over high heat.

2. Place the trimmed asparagus spears in a steamer basket and carefully lower it into the boiling water. Cover the pot with a lid.

3. Steam the asparagus for 5-7 minutes, or until it is tender-crisp.

4. Carefully remove the steamer basket from the pot and transfer the asparagus to a serving dish.

5. Drizzle the asparagus with the olive oil and sprinkle with the lemon zest and lemon juice. Toss gently to coat.

6. Season the steamed asparagus with salt and pepper to taste. Serve the asparagus warm or at room temperature.

This simple steamed asparagus dish is an excellent choice for a menopause-friendly diet. Asparagus is a nutrient-dense vegetable that is high in folate, fiber, and antioxidants, which can help support overall health during this transition.

The lemon zest and juice provide a bright, refreshing flavor and a boost of vitamin C. The olive oil adds healthy fats that can help reduce inflammation.

This side dish is easy to prepare and pairs well with a variety of main courses, such as grilled fish, roasted chicken, or vegetarian options. Enjoy the delicious and nutritious combination of steamed asparagus and lemon zest.

How would you rate this dish?

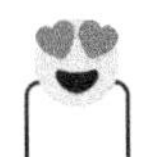 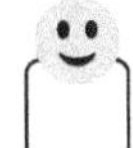 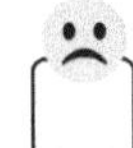 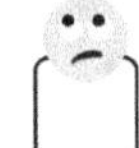 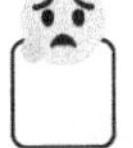

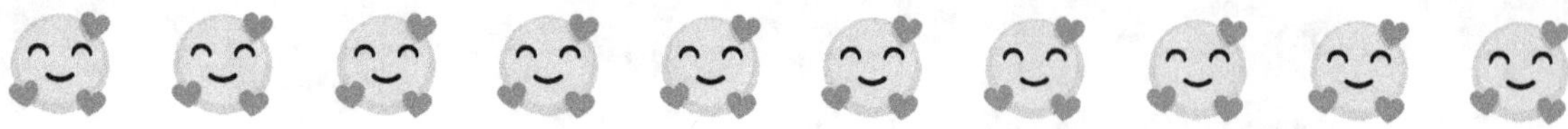

95. Sweet Potato Fries with Paprika

 Prep Time :   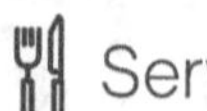 Cook Time :   Servings :

Let's do that and fill in the time here

Is this dish easy or difficult for you to make?

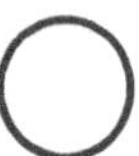 ◯    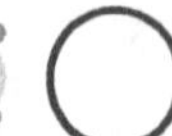 ◯

Write 5 friends with whom you want to share this dish

INGREDIENTS

- 2 large sweet potatoes, peeled and cut into 1/2-inch thick fries
- 2 tbsp olive oil
- 1 tsp paprika
- 1/2 tsp garlic powder
- 1/4 tsp salt
- 1/4 tsp black pepper

1. Preheat oven to 400°F. Line a baking sheet with parchment paper.

2. In a large bowl, toss the sweet potato fries with the olive oil, paprika, garlic powder, salt, and pepper until evenly coated.

3. Spread the fries in a single layer on the prepared baking sheet.

4. Bake for 20-25 minutes, flipping halfway, until the fries are crispy and lightly browned. Serve hot.

Why this is a good menopause diet option:

- Sweet potatoes are a great source of fiber, vitamins, and minerals that can help support overall health during menopause.

- The healthy fats from the olive oil provide anti-inflammatory benefits.

- Spices like paprika and garlic powder add flavor without needing to use a lot of salt.

- Baking the fries instead of frying keeps them lower in calories and unhealthy fats.

This recipe is simple, nutritious, and can be a tasty side dish or snack option for women going through menopause.

How would you rate this dish?

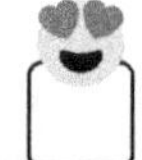 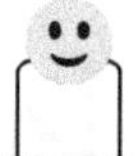 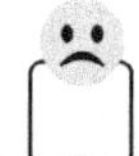 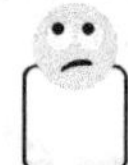 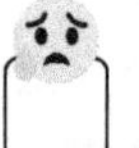

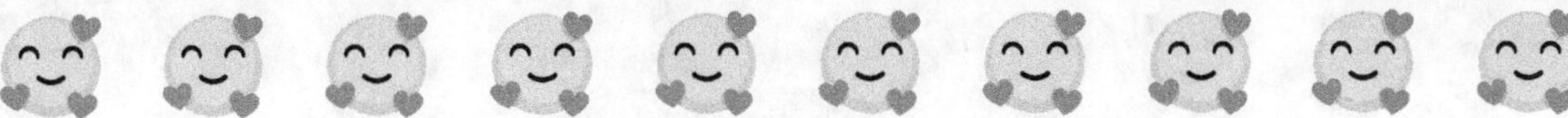

96. Sautéed Spinach with Garlic

 Prep Time :

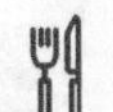 Cook Time :

Servings :

Write 5 friends with whom you want to share this dish

....
....
....
....
....

Is this dish easy or difficult for you to make?

 ◯   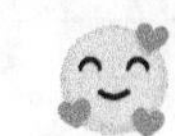 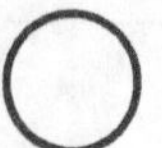 ◯

INGREDIENTS

- 1 lb fresh spinach, washed and stems removed
- 2 tbsp olive oil
- 3 cloves garlic, minced
- 1/4 tsp red pepper flakes (optional)
- Salt and pepper to taste

1. Heat the olive oil in a large skillet or wok over medium heat. Add the minced garlic and red pepper flakes (if using) and cook for 1 minute, stirring constantly, until fragrant.

2. Add the spinach to the skillet in batches, stirring constantly, until the spinach is wilted down, about 2-3 minutes per batch.

3. Once all the spinach is wilted, season with salt and pepper to taste.

4. Serve the sautéed spinach immediately, while hot. Enjoy!

The key is to sauté the spinach quickly over high heat to wilt it down without overcooking. The garlic and optional red pepper flakes add great flavor. This makes a simple, healthy side dish that pairs well with many main courses.

How would you rate this dish?

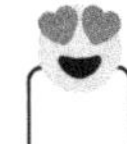 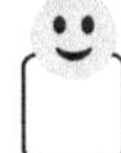  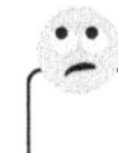 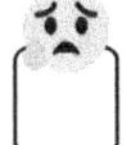

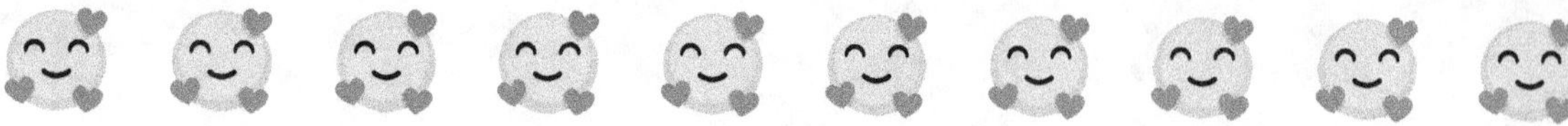

97. Roasted Carrots with Honey and Thyme

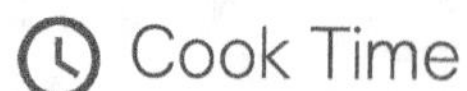 Prep Time :   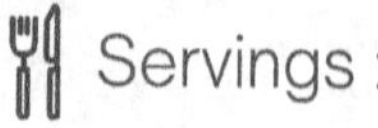 Cook Time :   Servings :

Write 5 friends with whom you want to share this dish

....
....
....
....
....

Is this dish easy or difficult for you to make?

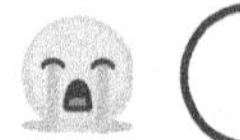 ○    ○

INGREDIENTS

- 1 lb carrots, peeled and cut into 1-inch pieces
- 2 tbsp olive oil
- 2 tbsp honey
- 1 tsp fresh thyme leaves (or 1/2 tsp dried thyme)
- Salt and pepper to taste

1. Preheat your oven to 400°F (200°C).

2. In a large bowl, toss the carrot pieces with the olive oil, honey, thyme, salt, and pepper until the carrots are evenly coated.

3. Spread the carrots out in a single layer on a baking sheet lined with parchment paper.

4. Roast the carrots for 20-25 minutes, stirring halfway, until they are tender and lightly caramelized.

5. Serve the roasted carrots warm, garnished with any extra thyme leaves if desired.

This dish is perfect for a menopause diet for a few reasons:

- Carrots are a great source of beta-carotene, which can help support skin and eye health during menopause.
- Honey provides a natural sweetness without the blood sugar spike of refined sugar.
- Thyme is an herb that has anti-inflammatory properties, which can help manage menopausal symptoms.
- The dish is low in calories and fat, making it a healthy side option.

Enjoy this simple yet flavorful roasted carrot recipe as part of a balanced menopause-friendly meal.

How would you rate this dish?

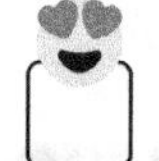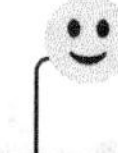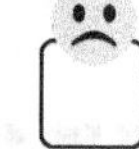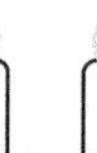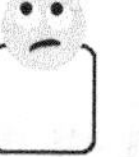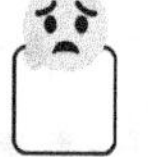

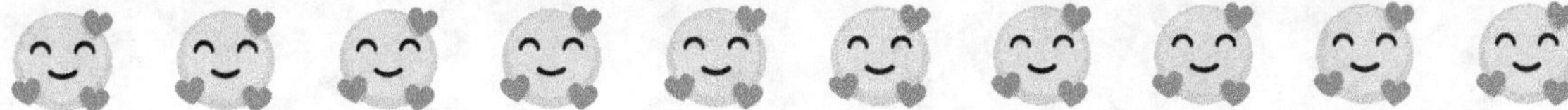

98. Broccoli with Lemon and Parmesan

 Prep Time :   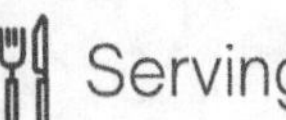 Cook Time :   Servings :

Is this dish easy or difficult for you to make?

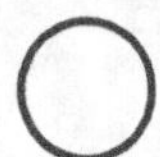 ◯   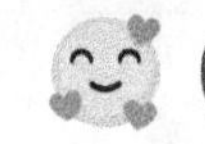 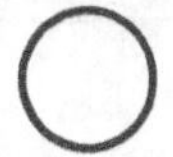 ◯

Write 5 friends with whom you want to share this dish ....

INGREDIENTS

- 3 medium zucchini, spiralized or julienned into noodles
- 1/2 cup fresh basil leaves
- 1/4 cup pine nuts
- 2 cloves garlic
- 2 tablespoons olive oil
- 2 tablespoons grated Parmesan cheese
- 1 tablespoon lemon juice
- Salt and pepper to taste

How would you rate this dish?

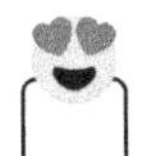 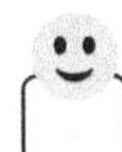 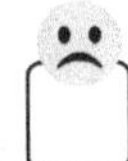 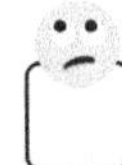 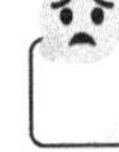

1. In a food processor or blender, combine the fresh basil leaves, pine nuts, and garlic. Pulse until finely chopped.

2. Add the olive oil, Parmesan cheese, and lemon juice. Blend until a smooth pesto sauce forms. Season with salt and pepper to taste.

3. In a large skillet or wok, heat the zucchini noodles over medium heat for 2-3 minutes, just until they start to soften slightly. Be careful not to overcook them.

4. Remove the zucchini noodles from heat and toss them with the prepared pesto sauce until evenly coated.

5. Serve the zucchini noodles with pesto immediately, garnished with additional Parmesan cheese or pine nuts if desired.

This zucchini noodle dish is an excellent choice for a menopause-friendly diet. Zucchini is a low-calorie, fiber-rich vegetable that can help support digestive health. The pesto sauce is made with nutrient-dense ingredients like basil, pine nuts, and Parmesan cheese.

The healthy fats from the olive oil and pine nuts can help reduce inflammation, while the lemon juice provides a boost of vitamin C. This dish is a delicious and nutritious way to incorporate more plant-based foods into your diet during menopause.

Enjoy this flavorful and satisfying zucchini noodle dish as a main course or a side to grilled protein.

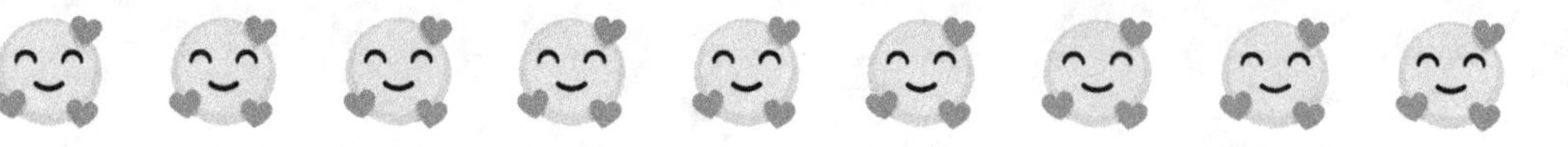

99. Cauliflower Rice with Herbs

 Prep Time : 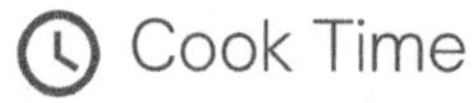 Cook Time :  Servings :

Is this dish easy or difficult for you to make?

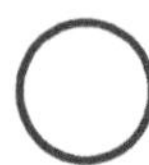 ○   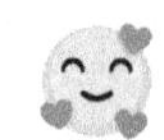 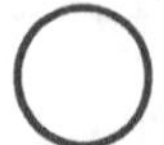 ○

Write 5 friends with whom you want to share this dish

....
....
....
....
....
....

INGREDIENTS

- 1 head of cauliflower, cut into florets
- 2 tbsp olive oil
- 2 cloves garlic, minced
- 2 tbsp chopped fresh herbs (such as parsley, basil, or cilantro)
- Salt and pepper to taste

1. In a food processor, pulse the cauliflower florets until they resemble the size and texture of rice grains. Be careful not to over-process.

2. In a large skillet, heat the olive oil over medium heat. Add the minced garlic and sauté for 1-2 minutes until fragrant.

3. Add the riced cauliflower to the skillet and sauté for 5-7 minutes, stirring occasionally, until the cauliflower is tender and lightly browned.

4. Remove the skillet from heat and stir in the chopped fresh herbs. Season with salt and pepper to taste.

5. Serve the cauliflower rice warm, as a side dish or as a base for other dishes.

Benefits for Menopause:

1. Low-Carb: Cauliflower rice is a low-carb, low-calorie alternative to traditional rice, making it a great option for maintaining a healthy weight during menopause.

2. Fiber: Cauliflower is a good source of fiber, which can help with digestive issues that may arise during menopause.

3. Antioxidant Support: Cauliflower is rich in antioxidants, such as vitamin C and carotenoids, which can help combat oxidative stress associated with menopause.

How would you rate this dish?

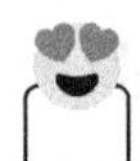 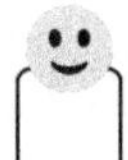 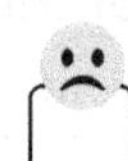 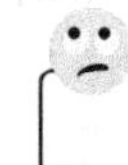 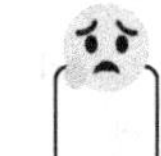

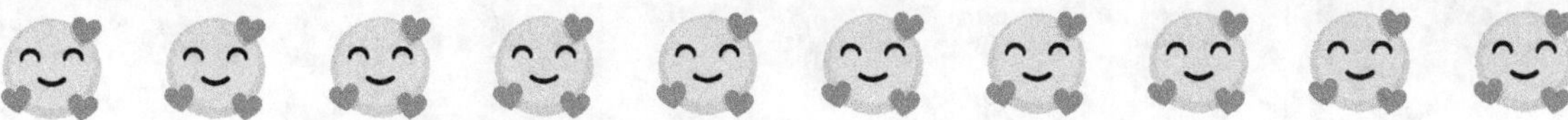

100. Zucchini Noodles with Pesto

 *Let's do that and fill in the time here* 

Prep Time :

Cook Time :

Servings :

Is this dish easy or difficult for you to make?

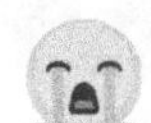  ◯   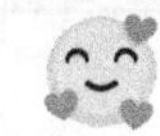  ◯

Write 5 friends with whom you want to share this dish

....

....

....

....

....

INGREDIENTS

- 3 medium zucchinis, spiralized or julienned into noodles
- 1/2 cup basil pesto (store-bought or homemade)
- 2 tbsp grated Parmesan cheese (optional)
- Salt and pepper to taste

1. Prepare the zucchini noodles by spiralizing or julienning the zucchinis. Set aside.

2. In a large bowl, toss the zucchini noodles with the basil pesto until the noodles are evenly coated.

3. If desired, sprinkle the grated Parmesan cheese over the top.

4. Season with salt and pepper to taste.

5. Serve the zucchini noodles with pesto immediately.

Benefits for Menopause:

1. Low-Calorie: Zucchini noodles are a low-calorie, low-carb alternative to traditional pasta, making them a great option for maintaining a healthy weight during menopause.

2. Hydration: Zucchinis are high in water content, which can help with hydration, a common issue during menopause.

3. Antioxidant Support: Zucchinis are a good source of antioxidants like vitamin C and carotenoids, which can help combat oxidative stress associated with menopause.

4. Bone Health: The basil in the pesto provides a source of vitamin K, which is important for maintaining bone density during the menopausal transition.

How would you rate this dish?

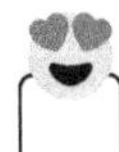 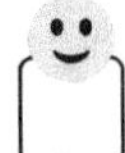  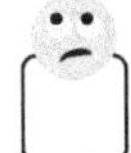 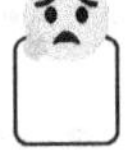

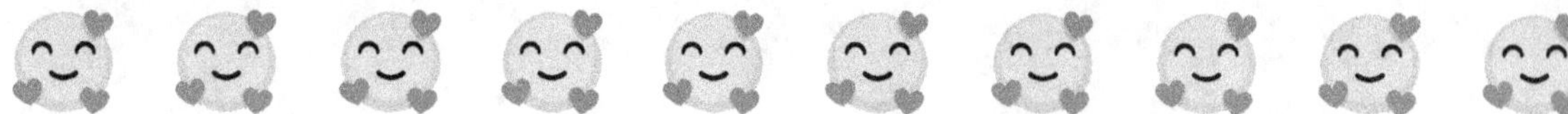

101. Green Tea with Lemon

 Prep Time :   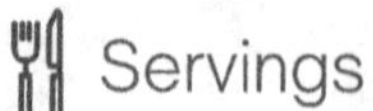 Cook Time :   Servings :

Is this dish easy or difficult for you to make?

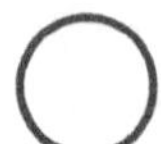 ◯    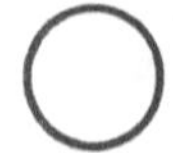 ◯

Write 5 friends with whom you want to share this dish

INGREDIENTS

- 1 cup hot water
- 1 green tea bag or 1-2 tsp loose leaf green tea
- 1 tbsp fresh lemon juice

1. Bring 1 cup of water to a boil.
2. Place the green tea bag or loose leaf tea in a mug.
3. Pour the hot water over the tea and let it steep for 3-5 minutes.
4. Remove the tea bag or strain the loose leaf tea.
5. Stir in the fresh lemon juice.

Benefits for Menopause:

1. Hydration: Green tea and lemon juice both contribute to overall hydration, which is important during menopause when dehydration can be a concern.

2. Antioxidant Support: Green tea is rich in antioxidants, such as polyphenols, that can help combat the oxidative stress associated with menopause.

3. Hormone Balance: Some studies suggest that the compounds in green tea may help regulate hormone levels and alleviate menopausal symptoms like hot flashes and mood swings.

4. Bone Health: Lemon is a good source of vitamin C, which is important for maintaining bone density during the menopausal transition.

5. Digestive Support: The citric acid in lemon can help stimulate digestive processes and may alleviate menopausal issues like bloating or constipation.

The combination of green tea and lemon provides a refreshing, slightly tart, and subtly sweet flavor that can be enjoyed hot or iced. You can adjust the amount of lemon juice to suit your taste preferences.

How would you rate this dish?

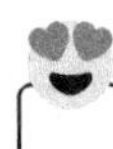 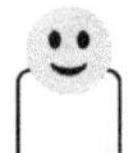 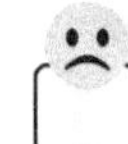 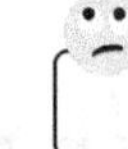 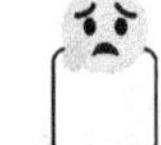

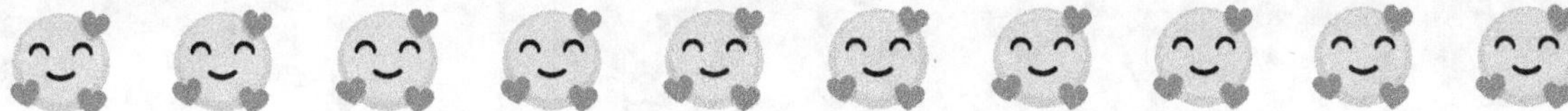

102. Herbal Tea with Mint

Let's do that and fill in the time here

Write 5 friends with whom you want to share this dish

....

....

....

....

....

INGREDIENTS

- 1 cup hot water
- 1-2 tsp dried peppermint leaves or 3-4 fresh mint leaves
- Honey or lemon (optional)

Is this dish easy or difficult for you to make?

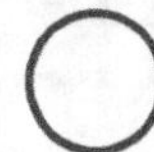 ◯   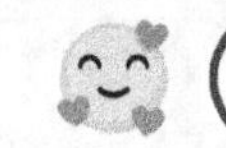 ◯

1. Bring 1 cup of water to a boil.
2. Place the dried peppermint leaves or fresh mint leaves in a mug or teapot.
3. Pour the hot water over the mint and let it steep for 5-7 minutes.
4. Strain the tea if using dried leaves.
5. Sweeten with a teaspoon of honey or a squeeze of lemon, if desired.

Benefits for Menopause:

1. Soothing Digestion: Mint is known for its ability to soothe the digestive system, which can help alleviate common menopausal issues like bloating, gas, and constipation.

2. Reducing Hot Flashes: Mint contains menthol, which has a cooling effect that may help reduce the intensity and frequency of hot flashes.

3. Stress Relief: Mint has a calming aroma that can help reduce stress and anxiety, which are common during the menopausal transition.

4. Anti-Inflammatory Properties: Mint contains antioxidants and anti-inflammatory compounds that can help manage inflammation associated with menopause.

5. Hydration: Herbal tea is a great way to stay hydrated, which is important during menopause when dehydration can be a concern.

The simplicity of this herbal tea makes it an easy and versatile option for a menopause-friendly beverage. You can enjoy it hot or iced, and the addition of honey or lemon can provide extra flavor and health benefits.

How would you rate this dish?

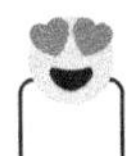 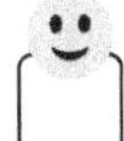 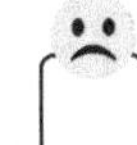 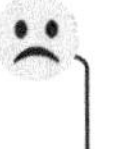 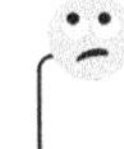 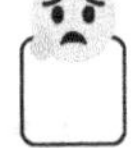

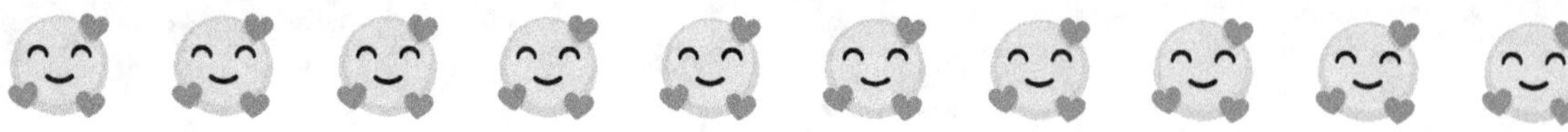

103. Water with Cucumber and Mint

Prep Time : 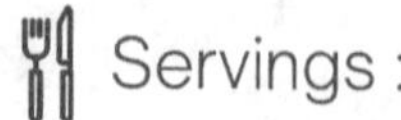

Cook Time :

Servings :

Is this dish easy or difficult for you to make?

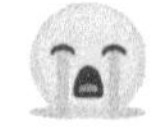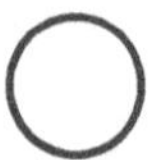 ◯   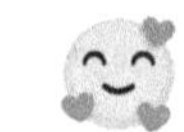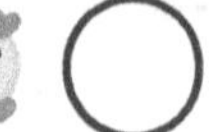 ◯

Write 5 friends with whom you want to share this dish

INGREDIENTS

- 4 cups water
- 1 cucumber, sliced
- 6-8 fresh mint leaves

1. In a pitcher, combine the water, cucumber slices, and mint leaves.
2. Refrigerate for at least 2 hours, or up to 24 hours, to allow the flavors to infuse.
3. Serve the cucumber mint water over ice.

Benefits for Menopause:

1. Hydration: Staying hydrated is crucial during menopause, and this infused water provides a refreshing way to increase fluid intake.

2. Cooling Properties: Cucumber and mint have a natural cooling effect, which can help alleviate menopausal symptoms like hot flashes and night sweats.

3. Digestive Support: Mint has anti-inflammatory properties and can help soothe the digestive system, which can be helpful for menopausal women experiencing issues like bloating or constipation.

4. Stress Reduction: The aroma of mint can have a calming effect, which may help reduce stress and anxiety, common during the menopausal transition.

5. Antioxidant Protection: Cucumbers contain antioxidants that can help combat the oxidative stress associated with menopause.

The combination of cucumber and mint provides a refreshing, subtly sweet, and slightly minty flavor that can be enjoyed throughout the day. You can adjust the amount of each ingredient to suit your taste preferences.

How would you rate this dish?

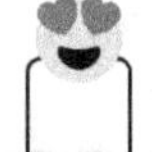 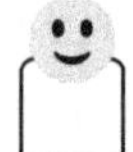 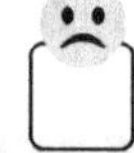 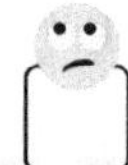 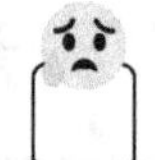

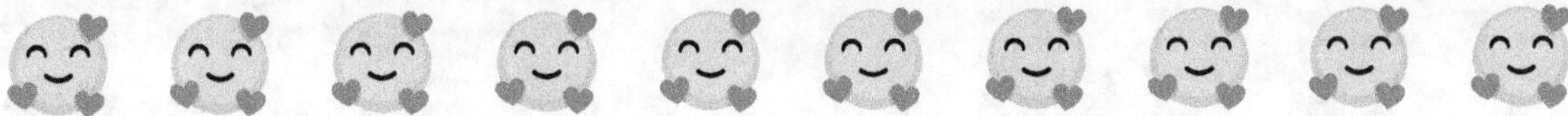
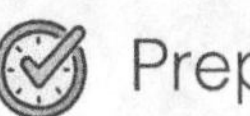 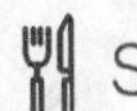

104. Coconut Water with Lime

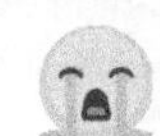 Prep Time :   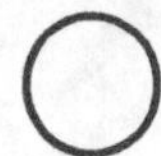 Cook Time :   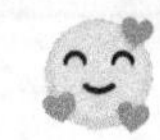 Servings :

Is this dish easy or difficult for you to make?

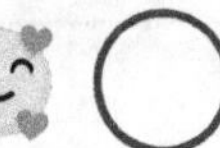 ◯   ◯

Write 5 friends with whom you want to share this dish

....
....
....
....
....

INGREDIENTS

- 1 cup unsweetened coconut water
- 1 tbsp fresh lime juice
- Ice (optional)

1. In a glass, combine the coconut water and lime juice. Stir to mix.
2. Add ice if desired.

Benefits for Menopause:

1. Hydration: Coconut water is an excellent source of natural electrolytes like potassium, which can help maintain proper hydration levels. Dehydration is common during menopause.

2. Bone Health: Coconut water contains small amounts of calcium, magnesium, and phosphorus, which are important minerals for maintaining bone health during menopause.

3. Antioxidant Support: Coconut water contains antioxidants like vitamin C, which can help combat oxidative stress and inflammation associated with menopause.

4. Hormone Balance: The potassium in coconut water may help regulate hormone levels and alleviate symptoms like hot flashes and mood swings.

5. Low Calorie: At just 46 calories per cup, coconut water is a low-calorie, hydrating beverage option that won't contribute to weight gain.

The addition of fresh lime juice provides a refreshing, tart flavor and a boost of vitamin C. This simple coconut water drink is a great way to stay hydrated and support your health during menopause.

How would you rate this dish?

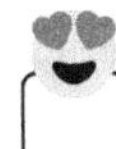 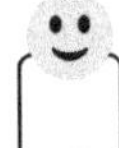 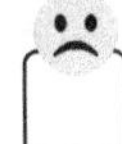 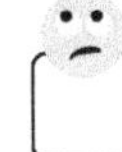 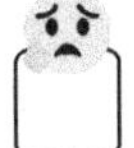

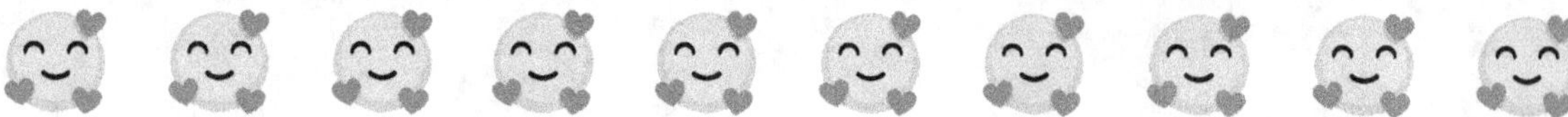

105. Homemade Iced Tea with Lemon

 *Let's do that and fill in the time here* Prep Time :   Cook Time :   Servings :

Write 5 friends with whom you want to share this dish

....
....
....
....
....

Is this dish easy or difficult for you to make?

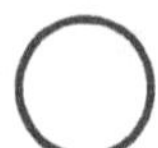 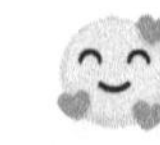 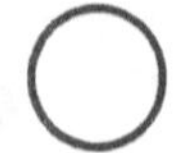 ◯   ◯

INGREDIENTS

- 4 cups water
- 4 black tea bags or 4 tsp loose leaf black tea
- 2 tbsp fresh lemon juice
- Honey or stevia (optional)

1. Bring the 4 cups of water to a boil in a saucepan.

2. Remove the water from heat and add the tea bags or loose leaf tea. Let it steep for 5-7 minutes.

3. Remove the tea bags or strain the loose leaf tea.

4. Stir in the fresh lemon juice and add honey or stevia to taste, if desired.

5. Pour the iced tea into a pitcher and refrigerate for at least 2 hours, or until chilled.. Serve the iced tea over ice.

Benefits for Menopause:

1. Hydration: Iced tea is a refreshing way to stay hydrated, which is crucial during menopause when dehydration can be a concern.

2. Antioxidant Support: Black tea is rich in antioxidants, such as polyphenols, that can help combat the oxidative stress associated with menopause.

3. Hormone Balance: The compounds in black tea may help regulate hormone levels and alleviate menopausal symptoms like hot flashes and mood swings.

4. Bone Health: Lemon is a good source of vitamin C, which is important for maintaining bone density during the menopausal transition.

How would you rate this dish?

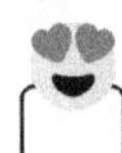 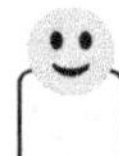 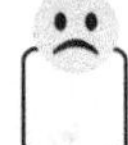 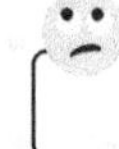 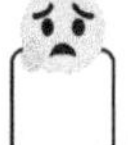

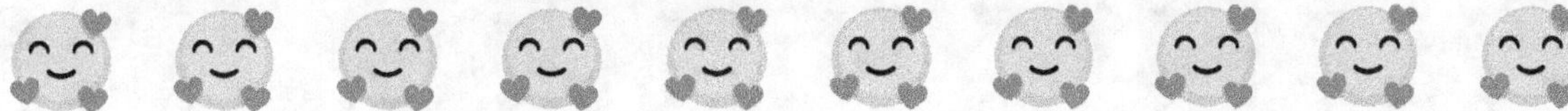

106. Almond Milk with Turmeric

 Prep Time :  Cook Time :   Servings :

Write 5 friends with whom you want to share this dish

....
....
....
....
....
....

Is this dish easy or difficult for you to make?

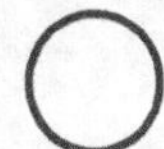 ◯    ◯

INGREDIENTS

- 4 cups unsweetened almond milk
- 1 tsp ground turmeric
- 1/2 tsp ground cinnamon (optional)
- 1 tbsp honey or maple syrup (optional)

1. In a saucepan, combine the almond milk, turmeric, and cinnamon (if using).
2. Heat the mixture over medium heat, stirring occasionally, until it's warm and the turmeric is fully dissolved, about 5 minutes.
3. Remove from heat and stir in the honey or maple syrup, if using.
4. Serve the almond milk with turmeric warm or chilled.

Benefits for Menopause:

1. Anti-Inflammatory Properties: Turmeric contains curcumin, a powerful anti-inflammatory compound that can help manage menopausal symptoms like joint pain and muscle aches.

2. Hormone Balance: Turmeric may help regulate hormone levels and alleviate symptoms like hot flashes and mood swings during menopause.

3. Bone Health: Almond milk is a good source of calcium, which is important for maintaining bone density during the menopausal transition.

4. Gut Health: The healthy fats in almond milk and the anti-inflammatory properties of turmeric can support a healthy gut microbiome, which is crucial for overall well-being during menopause.

5. Antioxidant Support: Both almond milk and turmeric are rich in antioxidants that can help combat the oxidative stress associated with menopause.

How would you rate this dish?

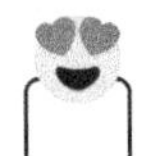 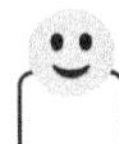 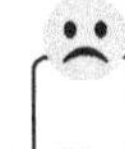 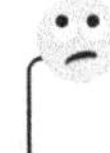 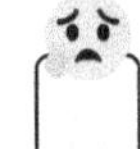

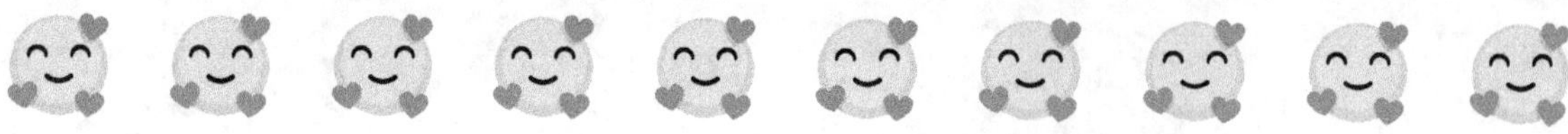

107. Berry Infused Water

Prep Time : 

Cook Time :

Servings : 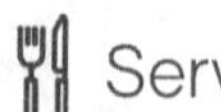

Is this dish easy or difficult for you to make?

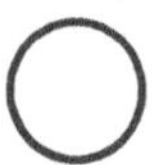 ◯ 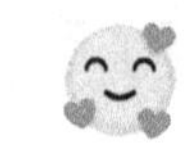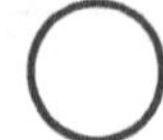 ◯

Write 5 friends with whom you want to share this dish

INGREDIENTS

- 4 cups water
- 1 cup mixed berries (such as raspberries, blueberries, and strawberries)
- 1 lemon, sliced (optional)

1. In a pitcher, combine the water and the mixed berries.

2. Refrigerate for at least 2 hours, or up to 24 hours, to allow the flavors to infuse.

3. Optionally, you can add sliced lemon to the pitcher for an extra burst of flavor.

4. Serve the berry infused water over ice.

Benefits for Menopause:

1. Antioxidant Support: Berries are rich in antioxidants, which can help combat the oxidative stress associated with menopause and support overall health.

2. Hormone Balance: Some studies suggest that certain berries, like blueberries, may help regulate hormone levels and alleviate menopausal symptoms like hot flashes and mood swings.

3. Bone Health: Berries, especially blackberries and raspberries, are a good source of vitamin C, which is important for maintaining bone density during the menopausal transition.

4. Hydration: Staying hydrated is crucial during menopause, and this infused water provides a refreshing way to increase fluid intake.

5. Gut Health: The natural prebiotic fibers in berries can help support a healthy gut microbiome, which is important for overall well-being during menopause.

How would you rate this dish?

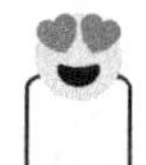 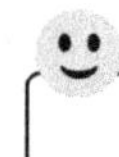 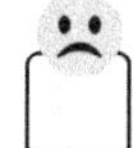 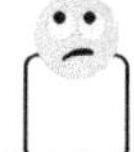 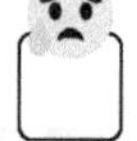

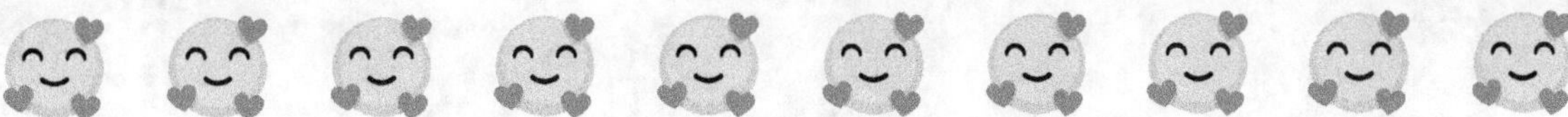

108. Lemon Ginger Water

Prep Time :   Cook Time :   Servings :

Is this dish easy or difficult for you to make?

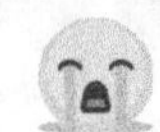 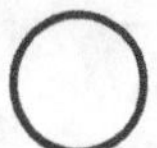 ◯   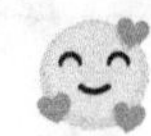  ◯

Write 5 friends with whom you want to share this dish

....
....
....
....
....

INGREDIENTS

- 4 cups water
- 1 lemon, sliced
- 1-inch piece of fresh ginger, sliced

1. In a pitcher, combine the water, lemon slices, and ginger slices.

2. Refrigerate for at least 2 hours, or up to 24 hours, to allow the flavors to infuse.

3. Serve the lemon ginger water over ice.

Benefits for Menopause:

1. Hydration: Staying hydrated is crucial during menopause, and this infused water provides a refreshing way to increase fluid intake.

2. Digestive Support: Ginger has anti-inflammatory properties and can help soothe the digestive system, which can be helpful for menopausal women experiencing issues like bloating or constipation.

3. Hormone Balance: Lemon contains citric acid, which may help balance hormone levels and alleviate symptoms like hot flashes and mood swings.

4. Antioxidant Protection: Both lemon and ginger are rich in antioxidants, which can help combat the oxidative stress associated with menopause.

5. Bone Health: Lemon is a good source of vitamin C, which is important for maintaining bone density during the menopausal transition.

The combination of lemon and ginger provides a refreshing, slightly tart, and subtly spicy flavor that can be enjoyed throughout the day. You can adjust the amount of each ingredient to suit your taste preferences.

How would you rate this dish?

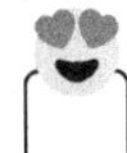 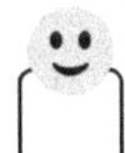  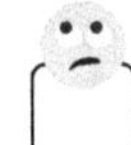 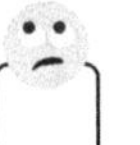 

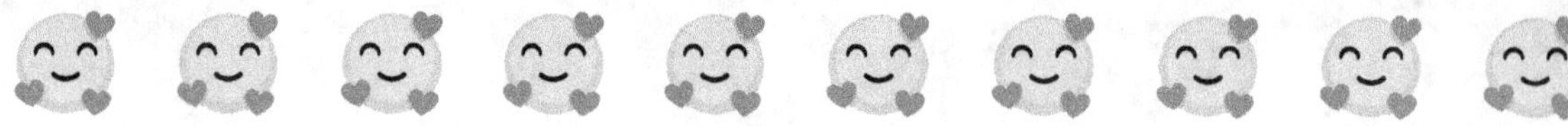

109. Chamomile Tea

Let's do that and fill in the time here

 Prep Time :   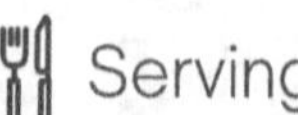 Cook Time :   Servings :

Write 5 friends with whom you want to share this dish

....

....

....

....

....

INGREDIENTS

- 1 cup hot water
- 1 chamomile tea bag or 1-2 tsp dried chamomile flowers

Is this dish easy or difficult for you to make?

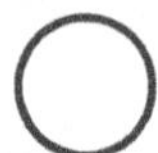 ◯   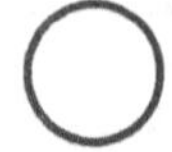 ◯

1. Bring 1 cup of water to a boil.
2. Place the chamomile tea bag or dried flowers in a mug.
3. Pour the hot water over the chamomile and let it steep for 5-7 minutes.
4. Remove the tea bag or strain the dried flowers.
5. Enjoy the chamomile tea warm or chilled.

Benefits for Menopause:

1. Stress and Anxiety Relief: Chamomile has been shown to have a calming effect and can help reduce stress and anxiety, which are common during the menopausal transition.

2. Improved Sleep: Chamomile tea may help promote better sleep, which can be challenging for many women going through menopause.

3. Reduced Inflammation: Chamomile contains anti-inflammatory compounds that can help alleviate menopausal symptoms like joint pain and muscle aches.

4. Digestive Support: Chamomile has soothing properties that can help with digestive issues like bloating or constipation, which can occur during menopause.

5. Antioxidant Protection: Chamomile is rich in antioxidants that can help combat the oxidative stress associated with menopause.

How would you rate this dish?

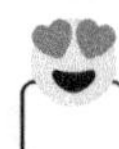 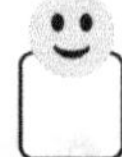 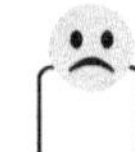 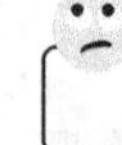 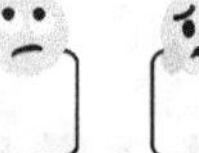 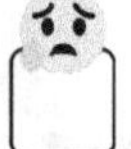

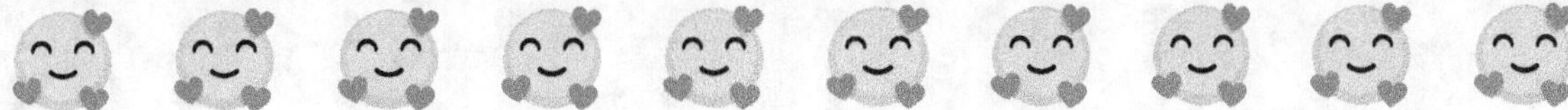

110. Apple Cider Vinegar Drink with Honey

 Prep Time :   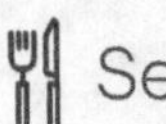 Cook Time :   Servings :

Write 5 friends with whom you want to share this dish

....
....
....
....
....

INGREDIENTS

- 1 tbsp apple cider vinegar
- 1 tbsp honey
- 1 cup warm water

Is this dish easy or difficult for you to make?

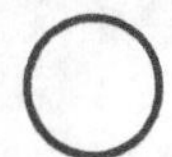 ◯    ◯

1. In a glass, combine the apple cider vinegar and honey.
2. Add the warm water and stir until the honey is fully dissolved.
3. Enjoy the drink warm or chilled.

Benefits for Menopause:

1. Blood Sugar Regulation: Apple cider vinegar can help regulate blood sugar levels, which is important during menopause when hormonal changes can affect insulin sensitivity.

2. Gut Health: The acetic acid in apple cider vinegar can help promote a healthy gut microbiome, which is crucial for overall well-being during menopause.

3. Inflammation Reduction: Both apple cider vinegar and honey have anti-inflammatory properties that can help manage menopausal symptoms like joint pain and muscle aches.

4. Bone Health: Honey contains small amounts of minerals like calcium, magnesium, and phosphorus, which are important for maintaining bone density during menopause.

5. Hydration: The warm water in this drink can help keep you hydrated, which is essential during menopause when dehydration is common.

You can adjust the ratios of apple cider vinegar and honey to suit your taste preferences. Start with 1 tbsp of each and gradually increase or decrease the amounts as needed.

How would you rate this dish?

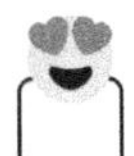 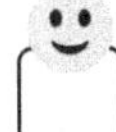  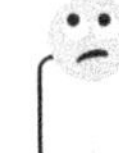 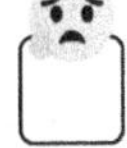

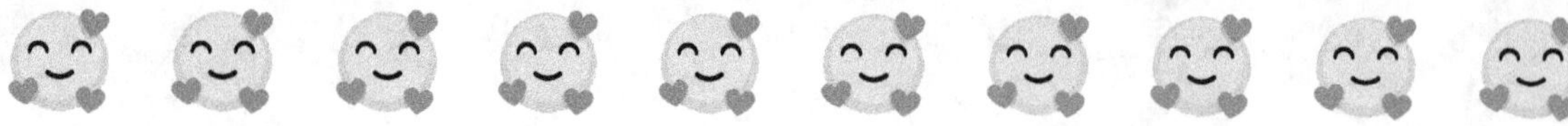

111. Homemade Trail Mix with Nuts and Dried Fruits

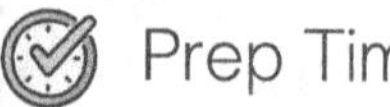 Prep Time :    Cook Time :   Servings :

Is this dish easy or difficult for you to make?

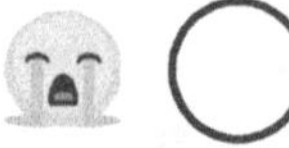 ◯    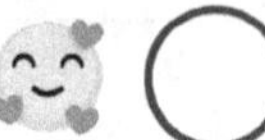 ◯

Write 5 friends with whom you want to share this dish

....

....

....

....

....

INGREDIENTS

- 1 cup raw almonds
- 1/2 cup raw walnuts
- 1/2 cup raw cashews
- 1/2 cup unsweetened dried cranberries
- 1/2 cup unsweetened dried apricots, chopped
- 1/4 cup unsweetened shredded coconut

1. In a large bowl, combine all the ingredients and mix well.
2. Store the trail mix in an airtight container at room temperature.

Benefits for Menopause:

1. Healthy Fats: The nuts in the trail mix provide healthy monounsaturated and polyunsaturated fats, which can help support hormone balance and reduce inflammation during menopause.

2. Protein: The nuts and dried fruits offer a good source of plant-based protein, which is important for maintaining muscle mass and bone health during the menopausal transition.

3. Antioxidant Support: The dried fruits, such as cranberries and apricots, are rich in antioxidants that can help combat the oxidative stress associated with menopause.

4. Bone Health: The nuts, especially almonds and walnuts, contain minerals like calcium, magnesium, and phosphorus, which are essential for maintaining strong bones during menopause.

5. Fiber: The combination of nuts and dried fruits provides a good source of fiber, which can help with digestive issues that may arise during menopause.

This homemade trail mix is a versatile, nutrient-dense snack that can be enjoyed throughout the day. You can customize the ingredients to your taste preferences, such as adding different types of nuts or dried fruits.

How would you rate this dish?

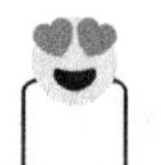 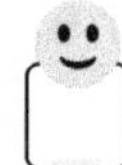 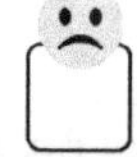 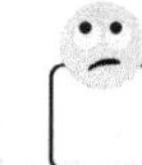 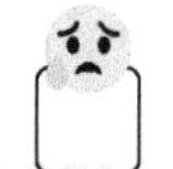

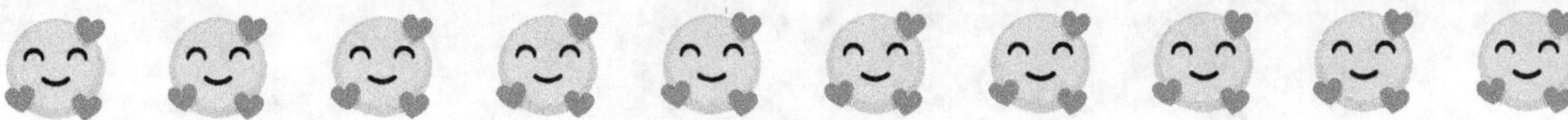

112. Baked Kale Chips

🕐 Prep Time :   🕐 Cook Time :   🍴 Servings :

Is this dish easy or difficult for you to make?

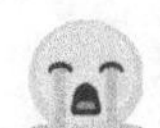 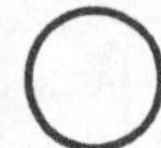 ◯   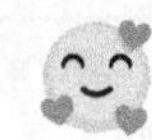 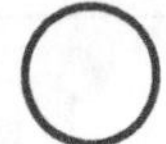 ◯

Write 5 friends with whom you want to share this dish

....
....
....
....
....

INGREDIENTS

- 1 bunch of kale, stems removed and leaves torn into bite-sized pieces
- 1-2 tbsp olive oil
- Salt and pepper to taste

1. Preheat your oven to 350°F (175°C).

2. Wash and thoroughly dry the kale leaves. Place them in a large bowl.

3. Drizzle the kale with olive oil and toss to coat the leaves evenly.

4. Spread the kale leaves in a single layer on a baking sheet lined with parchment paper.

5. Bake for 12-15 minutes, flipping the leaves halfway, until they are crispy and lightly browned.

6. Remove the kale chips from the oven and season with salt and pepper to taste. Serve the baked kale chips immediately.nefits for Menopause:

1. Nutrient-Dense: Kale is packed with vitamins, minerals, and antioxidants, including vitamins A, C, and K, as well as calcium and magnesium, which are important during menopause.

2. Anti-Inflammatory Properties: Kale contains anti-inflammatory compounds that can help manage menopausal symptoms like joint pain and muscle aches.

3. Bone Health: The calcium and vitamin K in kale contribute to maintaining strong bones during the menopausal transition.

4. Gut Health: Kale is a good source of fiber, which can help support a healthy gut microbiome, crucial for overall well-being during menopause.

How would you rate this dish?

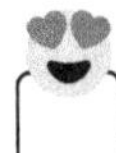 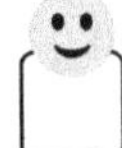 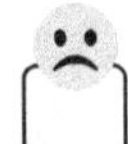 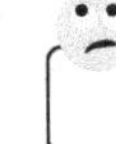 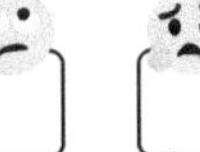 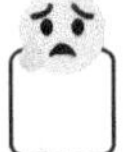

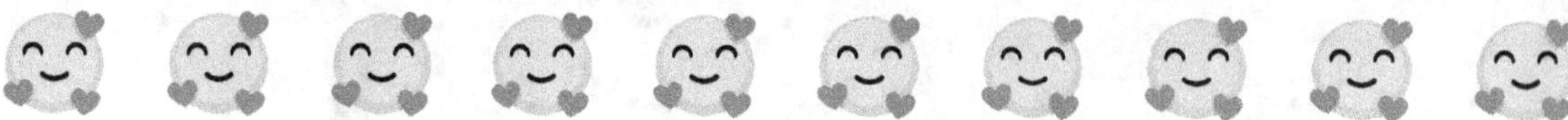

113. Stuffed Avocados with Tuna Salad

Let's do that and fill in the time here Prep Time :   Cook Time :   Servings :

Write 5 friends with whom you want to share this dish

....
....
....
....
....

INGREDIENTS

- 2 ripe avocados, halved and pitted
- 1 (5 oz) can of tuna, drained
- 2 tbsp plain Greek yogurt
- 1 tbsp lemon juice
- 1 tbsp finely chopped celery
- 1 tbsp finely chopped red onion
- 1 tsp Dijon mustard
- Salt and pepper to taste

Is this dish easy or difficult for you to make?

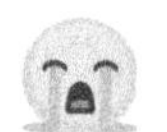 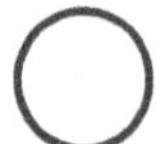 ○   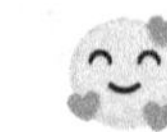  ○

1. In a medium bowl, mix together the tuna, Greek yogurt, lemon juice, celery, red onion, and Dijon mustard. Season with salt and pepper.
2. Scoop the tuna salad mixture into the avocado halves, dividing it evenly.
3. Serve the stuffed avocados immediately.

Benefits for Menopause:

1. Healthy Fats: Avocados are rich in monounsaturated fats, which can help support hormone balance and reduce inflammation during menopause.

2. Protein: The tuna provides a good source of lean protein, which is important for maintaining muscle mass and bone health during the menopausal transition.

3. Antioxidant Support: Avocados are a great source of antioxidants, such as vitamin C and carotenoids, that can help combat the oxidative stress associated with menopause.

4. Bone Health: Avocados and tuna both contain nutrients like calcium, magnesium, and vitamin D, which are essential for maintaining strong bones during menopause.

5. Digestive Support: The Greek yogurt in the tuna salad can help promote a healthy gut microbiome, which is crucial for overall well-being during menopause.

How would you rate this dish?

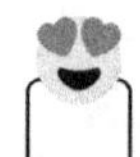 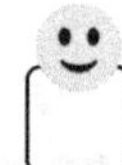 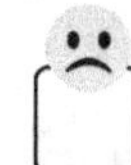 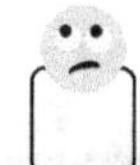 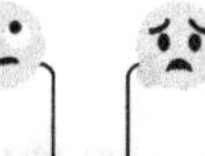

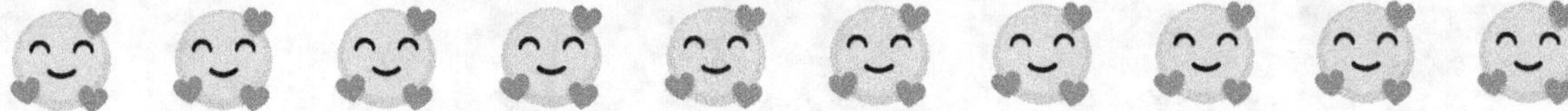

114. Cucumber Slices with Greek Yogurt Dip

 Prep Time :   Cook Time :   Servings :

Write 5 friends with whom you want to share this dish

....

....

....

....

....

Is this dish easy or difficult for you to make?

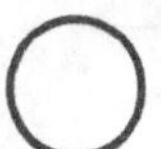 ○   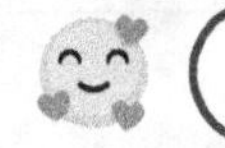 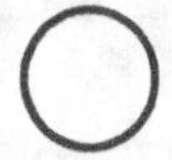 ○

INGREDIENTS

- 1 large cucumber, sliced into rounds or spears
- 1 cup plain Greek yogurt
- 1 tbsp fresh dill, chopped
- 1 tbsp lemon juice
- 1 clove garlic, minced
- Salt and pepper to taste

1. In a small bowl, mix together the Greek yogurt, dill, lemon juice, and minced garlic. Season with salt and pepper to taste.
2. Arrange the cucumber slices or spears on a serving platter.
3. Serve the Greek yogurt dip alongside the cucumber slices.

Benefits for Menopause:

1. Hydration: Cucumbers are high in water content, which can help with hydration, a common issue during menopause.

2. Bone Health: Greek yogurt is a good source of calcium, which is important for maintaining bone density during the menopausal transition.

3. Gut Health: The probiotics in Greek yogurt can help support a healthy gut microbiome, which is crucial for overall well-being during menopause.

4. Anti-Inflammatory Properties: Cucumbers contain antioxidants and anti-inflammatory compounds that can help manage menopausal symptoms like joint pain and muscle aches.

5. Hormone Balance: The combination of healthy fats from the yogurt and the phytonutrients in the cucumbers may help support hormone balance and alleviate symptoms like hot flashes and mood swings.

This simple, refreshing snack is a great way to incorporate more vegetables and dairy into your menopause diet. You can customize the dip by adding different herbs or spices to suit your taste preferences

How would you rate this dish?

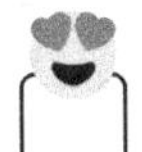  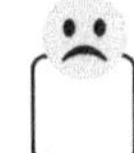 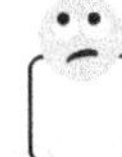 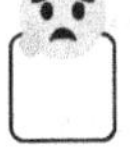

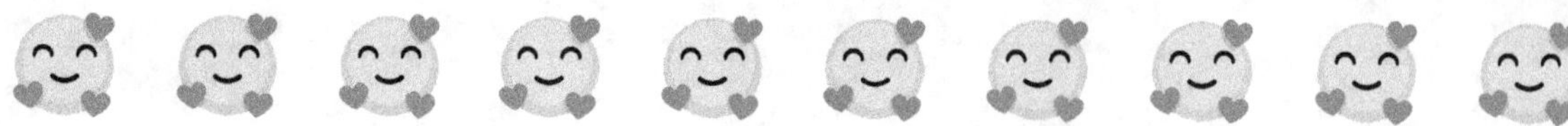

115. Whole Grain Toast with Mashed Avocado and Tomato

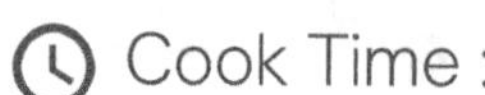 Prep Time :   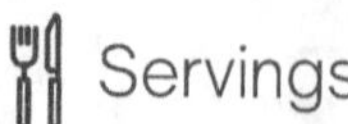 Cook Time :   Servings :

Is this dish easy or difficult for you to make?

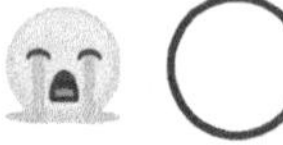 ◯   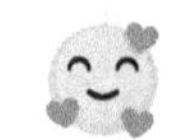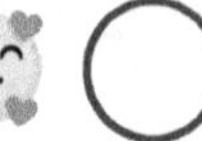 ◯

Write 5 friends with whom you want to share this dish

....

....

....

....

....

INGREDIENTS

- 2 slices of whole grain bread
- 1 ripe avocado, mashed
- 1 tomato, sliced
- Salt and pepper to taste

1. Toast the whole grain bread until lightly golden.
2. Spread the mashed avocado evenly over the toasted bread slices.
3. Top the avocado with sliced tomatoes.
4. Season with salt and pepper to taste.

Benefits for Menopause:

1. Healthy Fats: Avocado is rich in monounsaturated fats, which can help support hormone balance and reduce inflammation during menopause.

2. Fiber and Antioxidants: Whole grain bread, avocado, and tomatoes provide a good source of fiber and antioxidants that can help combat the oxidative stress associated with menopause.

3. Bone Health: Avocado and whole grains contain important minerals like calcium, magnesium, and phosphorus, which are essential for maintaining strong bones during the menopausal transition.

4. Digestive Support: The fiber in the whole grain bread and the healthy fats in the avocado can help promote a healthy gut microbiome, which is crucial for overall well-being during menopause.

5. Hydration: Tomatoes are a good source of water, which can help with hydration, a common issue during menopause.

This simple, open-faced sandwich is a nutrient-dense and satisfying option that can be enjoyed for breakfast, lunch, or a snack. You can customize the toppings by adding other vegetables, herbs, or a sprinkle of feta cheese.

How would you rate this dish?

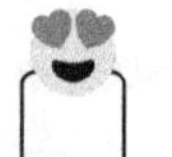 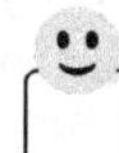 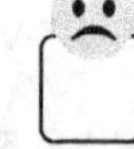 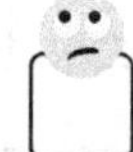 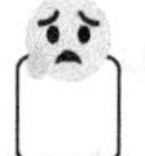

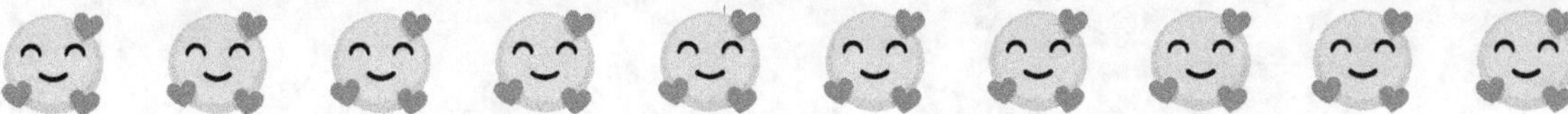

116. Roasted Chickpeas with Spices

*Let's do that and
fill in the time here*

 Prep Time :   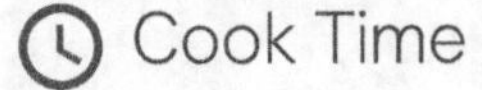 Cook Time :   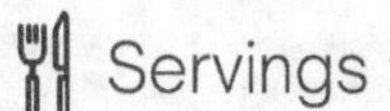 Servings :

Is this dish easy or difficult for you to make?

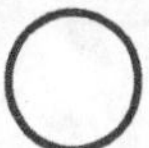 ◯   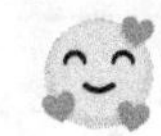 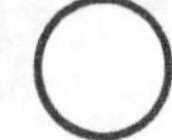 ◯

Write 5 friends with whom you want to share this dish

....

....

....

....

....

INGREDIENTS

- 1 (15 oz) can of chickpeas, drained and rinsed
- 1 tbsp olive oil
- 1 tsp ground cumin
- 1 tsp paprika
- 1/2 tsp garlic powder
- 1/4 tsp cayenne pepper (optional)
- Salt and pepper to taste

1. Preheat your oven to 400°F (200°C).
2. Pat the chickpeas dry with a paper towel to remove any excess moisture.
3. In a bowl, toss the chickpeas with the olive oil, cumin, paprika, garlic powder, and cayenne pepper (if using). Season with salt and pepper.
4. Spread the seasoned chickpeas in a single layer on a baking sheet.
5. Roast for 20-25 minutes, stirring halfway, until the chickpeas are crispy.
6. Remove the roasted chickpeas from the oven and let them cool slightly before serving.

Benefits for Menopause:

1. Protein and Fiber: Chickpeas are a good source of plant-based protein and fiber, which can help support satiety and maintain muscle mass during menopause.

2. Bone Health: Chickpeas contain calcium, magnesium, and other minerals that are important for maintaining strong bones during the menopausal transition.

3. Anti-Inflammatory Properties: The spices used in this recipe, such as cumin and paprika, have anti-inflammatory properties that can help manage menopausal symptoms like joint pain and muscle aches.

4. Antioxidant Support: Chickpeas and the spices used in this recipe are rich in antioxidants that can help combat the oxidative stress associated with menopause.

How would you rate this dish?

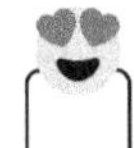  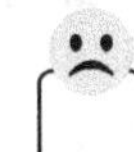 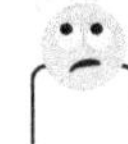 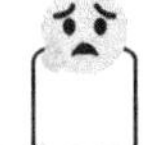

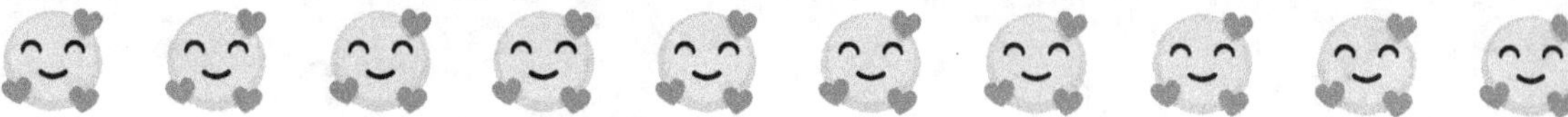

117. Boiled Eggs with Avocado

 Prep Time :  Cook Time : Servings :

Is this dish easy or difficult for you to make?

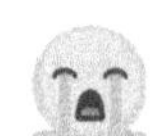 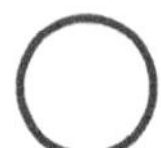 ◯    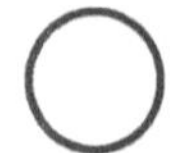 ◯

Write 5 friends with whom you want to share this dish

INGREDIENTS

- 2 hard-boiled eggs
- 1/2 ripe avocado, sliced or mashed
- Salt and pepper to taste

1. Prepare the hard-boiled eggs according to your preferred method.
2. Peel the eggs and slice them in half, or leave them whole.
3. Arrange the boiled egg halves or whole eggs on a plate.
4. Top the eggs with sliced or mashed avocado.
5. Season with salt and pepper to taste.

Benefits for Menopause:

1. Protein and Healthy Fats: The combination of eggs and avocado provides a balanced source of protein and healthy monounsaturated fats, which can help support hormone balance and reduce inflammation during menopause.

2. Bone Health: Eggs are a good source of vitamin D, while avocados contain calcium and other minerals essential for maintaining strong bones during the menopausal transition.

3. Antioxidant Support: Avocados are rich in antioxidants, such as vitamin C and carotenoids, that can help combat the oxidative stress associated with menopause.

4. Digestive Support: The healthy fats and fiber in avocados can help promote a healthy gut microbiome, which is crucial for overall well-being during menopause.

5. Satiety: The protein and healthy fats in this snack can help keep you feeling full and satisfied, which can be beneficial for managing weight during menopause.

How would you rate this dish?

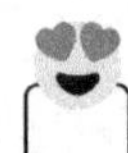 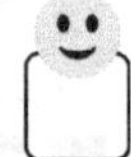 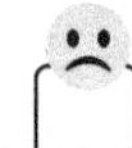 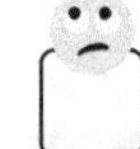 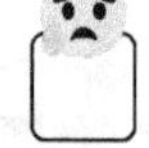

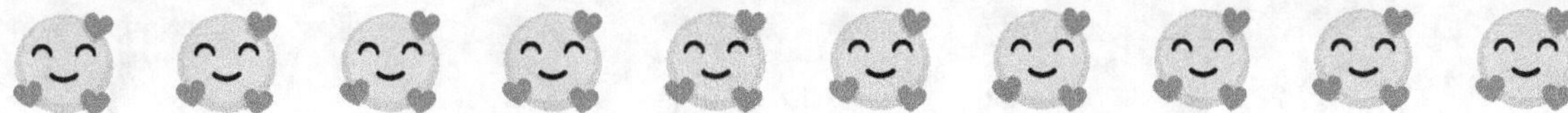

118. Homemade Vegetable Chips

 Prep Time :   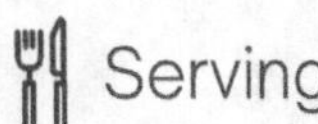 Cook Time :   Servings :

Is this dish easy or difficult for you to make?

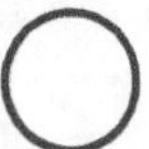 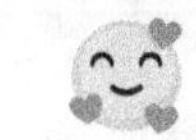 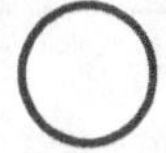

Write 5 friends with whom you want to share this dish

INGREDIENTS

- 1 lb mixed vegetables (such as thinly sliced zucchini, sweet potato, beets, or kale leaves)
- 1-2 tbsp olive oil or avocado oil
- Salt and pepper to taste

1. Preheat your oven to 350°F (175°C).
2. Wash and thoroughly dry the vegetable slices.
3. Arrange the vegetable slices in a single layer on baking sheets lined with parchment paper.
4. Brush or drizzle the vegetable slices with the oil, making sure they are evenly coated.
5. Sprinkle with salt and pepper to taste.
6. Bake for 15-25 minutes, flipping the slices halfway, until they are crispy and lightly browned.
7. Remove the vegetable chips from the oven and let them cool completely before serving.

Benefits for Menopause:

1. Nutrient-Dense: Vegetables like zucchini, sweet potatoes, and beets are packed with vitamins, minerals, and antioxidants that can support overall health during menopause.

2. Anti-Inflammatory Properties: Many of the vegetables used in this recipe contain anti-inflammatory compounds that can help manage menopausal symptoms like joint pain and muscle aches.

3. Bone Health: Vegetables like sweet potatoes and leafy greens are good sources of calcium, magnesium, and other minerals essential for maintaining strong bones during the menopausal transition.

4. Gut Health: The fiber in these vegetable chips can help support a healthy gut microbiome, which is crucial for overall well-being during menopause.

How would you rate this dish?

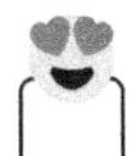 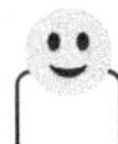 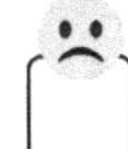 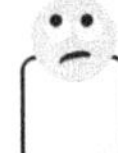 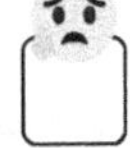

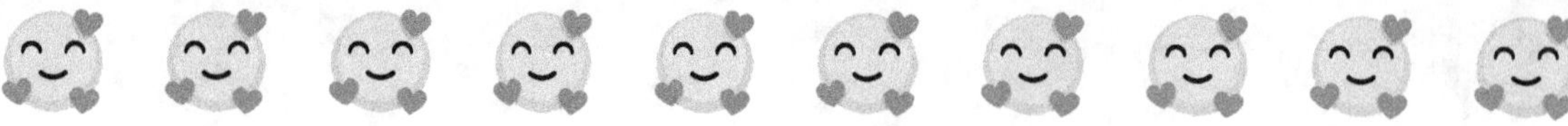

119. Yogurt Parfait with Granola and Berries

 Prep Time :

Cook Time :

Servings :

Is this dish easy or difficult for you to make?

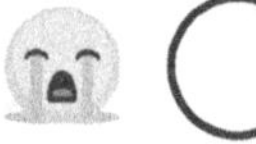 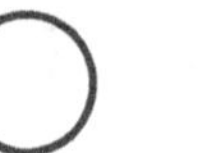 ◯    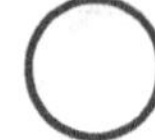 ◯

Write 5 friends with whom you want to share this dish

INGREDIENTS

- 1 cup plain Greek yogurt
- 1/2 cup fresh or frozen berries (such as blueberries, raspberries, or strawberries)
- 1/4 cup homemade or store-bought granola

1. In a glass or bowl, layer the yogurt, berries, and granola, repeating the layers until you reach the top.
2. Serve the yogurt parfait immediately.

Benefits for Menopause:

1. Protein and Calcium: The Greek yogurt provides a good source of protein and calcium, which are important for maintaining muscle mass and bone health during menopause.

2. Antioxidant Support: The berries are rich in antioxidants, such as vitamin C and anthocyanins, that can help combat the oxidative stress associated with menopause.

3. Fiber and Whole Grains: The granola adds fiber and whole grains, which can help with digestion and maintain a healthy gut microbiome during the menopausal transition.

4. Hormone Balance: The combination of protein, healthy fats, and complex carbohydrates in this parfait may help support hormone balance and alleviate menopausal symptoms like hot flashes and mood swings.

5. Hydration: The yogurt and berries contribute to overall hydration, which is crucial during menopause.

You can customize the parfait by using different types of berries or by making your own granola with nuts, seeds, and spices. This versatile and nutrient-dense breakfast or snack can be enjoyed throughout the day as part of a menopause-friendly diet.

How would you rate this dish?

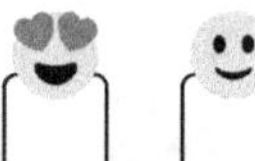 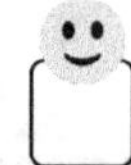 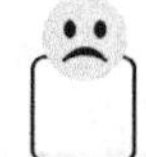 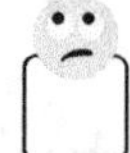 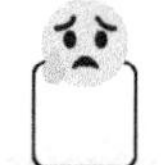

Congratulations on reaching the end of ***"The Good Food Menopause Diet Cookbook: A Comprehensive Guide to Flavorful Meals That Alleviate Menopause Symptoms and Promote Well-being."*** We hope this book has been a valuable resource, providing you with delicious recipes, essential nutritional information, and practical strategies to navigate menopause with confidence and ease.

Menopause is a significant life transition, and how you nourish your body during this time can make a profound difference in how you feel. By incorporating the recipes and dietary principles outlined in this book, you can alleviate many of the common symptoms associated with menopause, such as hot flashes, mood swings, and fatigue. More importantly, you can lay the foundation for long-term health and vitality.

Remember, the journey doesn't end here. The habits and choices you make today will continue to benefit you in the years to come. Here are a few key takeaways to keep in mind as you move forward:

1. Embrace Nutrient-Dense Foods: Focus on whole, unprocessed foods rich in essential nutrients that support hormonal balance and overall well-being.

2. Stay Hydrated: Drink plenty of water throughout the day to stay hydrated and help manage symptoms like hot flashes and dry skin.

3. Practice Mindful Eating: Pay attention to your body's hunger and fullness cues, and savor each bite to enhance your eating experience and improve digestion.

4. Stay Active: Complement your healthy eating habits with regular physical activity to boost your energy levels, maintain a healthy weight, and support bone health.

5. Listen to Your Body: Everyone's menopause experience is unique, so be attentive to how your body responds to different foods and adjust your diet accordingly.

As you continue on your menopause journey, remember that you have the power to make choices that enhance your quality of life. The recipes in this book are just the beginning—feel free to experiment, try new ingredients, and make these dishes your own. Cooking and eating should be enjoyable, and with the right approach, you can turn every meal into an opportunity to nurture your body and soul.

Thank you for allowing us to be a part of your menopause journey. We hope you find joy, comfort, and health in the meals you prepare and the lifestyle choices you make. Here's to a vibrant and fulfilling life during menopause and beyond!

Happy cooking and best wishes for your continued health and well-being.